Cover illustration:

Top: Freud's couch, brought with him from Vienna to London, where it now resides in the Freud Museum.

Bottom: A German fever thermometer from about 1920. Wagner-Jauregg won the Nobel Prize in 1927 by discovering that inducing malarial fevers in his patients reduced the ravages of neurosyphilis.

THE PSYCHOANALYST AND THE NAZI NOBELIST

THE CURIOUS STORY OF SIGMUND FREUD AND JULIUS WAGNER-JAUREGG

Wallace B. Mendelson

Pythagoras Press

Printed in the United States of America.

First printing: April 2022

ABOUT THE AUTHOR

Wallace Mendelson, MD is Professor of Psychiatry and Clinical Pharmacology (ret.) at the University of Chicago. He is a Distinguished Fellow of the American Psychiatric Association, and a member of the American Academy of Neuropsychopharmacology. He has been director of the Section on Sleep Studies at the National Institute of Mental Health, the Sleep Disorders Center at the Cleveland Clinic Foundation, and the Sleep Research Laboratory at the University of Chicago. He is the author of thirteen books and numerous professional papers. He is currently a Fellow of the Faculty of History and Philosophy of Medicine and Pharmacy at the Worshipful Society of Apothecaries, London. Among his honors have been the Academic Achievement Award from the American Sleep Disorders Association in 1999 and a special award for excellence in sleep and psychiatry from the National Sleep Foundation in 2010. More information about Dr. Mendelson's work is available in Wikipedia at https://en.wikipedia.org/wiki/Wallace_B._Mendelson and on his website at http://zhibit.org/wallacemendelson.

CONTENTS

PREFACE

Sigmund Freud and Julius Wagner-Jauregg were born and died within about a year of each other. They went to the same medical school, and afterwards studied neuropathology at the same institution. Both planned to go into internal medicine, and applied (unsuccessfully) for the same assistantships. They ultimately became brilliant physicians who contributed to the understanding of psychiatric conditions. Wagner-Jauregg was the first psychiatrist to win the Nobel Prize, for his febrile treatment of psychoses due to syphilis of the nervous system, while Freud developed the principles of psychoanalysis for treating mental disorders and understanding human behavior. Their last years, however, ended quite differently: Wagner-Jauregg became a Nazi supporter and advocate of 'racial hygiene', while Freud was terrorized by the Gestapo and had to flee to England.

Today, Freud's name is universally known, while few outside the specialty are familiar with Wagner-Jauregg. In the prologue of a previous book, *Trial by Fire,* I touched on the story of their interaction, and realized that it was something I wanted to come back to in more depth. Other psychiatrists and medical historians have tried to explain how these two extraordinary men turned out so differently, and how they were able to maintain a friendship, with birthday cards and correspondence using the German familiar word 'Du', rather than the more formal 'Sie'. Such works, however, are inevitably written for other scholars. I came to realize that this is too remarkable a piece of history to be confined to those with technical backgrounds. For this reason, I have tried to tell this story in a manner accessible to the general reader, and to emphasize not only the facts, but also what it was like to live at that time and to have the experiences which Freud and Wagner-Jauregg shared. It also speaks to topics we still consider, notably how we have come to treat mental illnesses with both 'talking therapies' and biological methods, though we are now learning that they are more similar than we might have supposed (Prosser et al., 2016).

The story of Wagner-Jauregg's discovery also touches on a second theme I've dwelt on in earlier writings—the remarkable interaction of the development of drugs for malaria and for psychiatric illness. *Molecules, Madness, and Malaria* (Mendelson, 2020) and the Appendix of this book describe how the rise of the synthetic fabric dye industry, beginning around the time of the birth of Freud and Wagner-Jauregg, evolved into the application of organic chemistry for making medicines. Among these were sulfa drugs for bacterial infections, antimalarials such as chloroquine, and later chlorpromazine, a failed antimalarial which revolutionized the treatment of psychoses in the 1950s. Malaria, then, interacted with the history of treating mental illness—first as an impetus for developing techniques for making medicines, and later, in the hands of Wagner-Jauregg, as a tool to produce fevers which treated syphilis of the nervous system in the years before the creation of penicillin. A few comments about how this book is set up: The first two chapters are summary biographies of Freud and Wagner-Jauregg, emphasizing the times at which their lives intersected, and pointing to where further information can be found later in the text. These are brief condensations for the purpose of providing a framework for understanding their interactions. The interested reader may wish to learn more in the detailed biographies of Freud by, for instance, Ernest Jones, Peter Gay or Joel Whitebook, and Wagner-Jauregg by Magda Whitrow. Here we are focused on only one aspect—but a remarkably fascinating one—of two complex lives.

Finally, I have tried to describe the interactions of these two figures in a narrative format, as much as possible as a continuous story which played out in their lives. In doing this, I was faced with the dilemma of how to provide background information which the general reader might find helpful, for instance the challenge of dementia paralytica to nineteenth century psychiatry, or how tuberculin was developed, or the manifestations of antisemitism in Austria at the time. In order to keep the flow of a narrative and not disrupt the story, this type of material is placed in an extensive Appendix, which is available to readers who would like to learn more about the context of the events portrayed here. The goal—and I hope you will find that I have achieved it—has been to find a balance which maintains the momentum of an evolving story while providing a framework of the environment in which it occurred.

REFERENCES for PREFACE

<u>Note:</u> *Regarding referencing throughout the book: In some cases, online materials do not provide a specific date of the original posting. In these situations, the year listed is the date the site was accessed.*

Gay, P. (ed), Freud, S. (author): *The Freud Reader*. W.W. Norton, 1995.
https://www.amazon.com/Freud-Reader-Sigmund/dp/0393314030/ref=sr_1_1?crid=WK07T6ZQO6UE&dchild=1&keywords=project+for+a+scientific+psychology+freud&qid=1611247644&sprefix=project+for+a+scientifi%2Caps%2C208&sr=8-1

Gay, P.: *Freud: A Life for Our Time* (New York: Norton, 1998), 448.

Jones, E. (author), Trilling, L. (ed.), and Marcus, S. (ed.): *The life and work of Sigmund Freud*. Plunket Lake Press, 2014.

Mendelson, W.B.: *Molecules, Madness, and Malaria: How Victorian Fabric Dyes Evolved into Modern Medicines for Mental Illness and Infectious Disease*. Pythagoras Press, 2020.
https://www.amazon.com/dp/B088QPG14K

Mendelson, W.B.: *Trial by Fire: World War II and the Founders of Modern Neuroscience and Psychopharmacology.* Pythagoras Press, 2021.
https://www.amazon.com/dp/B08X1MRVXJ

Prosser, A.; Helfer, B., and Leucht, S.: Biological V. Psychosocial treatments: a myth about pharmacotherapy v. psychotherapy. Brit. J. Psychiatry: the Journal of Mental Science. 208: 309-311, 2016.
https://www.researchgate.net/publication/299538003_Biological_V_Psychosocial_treatments_A_myth_about_pharmacotherapy_v_psychotherapy

Whitebook, J.: *Freud, an intellectual biography.* Cambridge University Press, 2017.

Whitrow, M.: Freud and Wagner-Jauregg: A historiographical study. Psychiatric Bulletin 14: 356-358, 1990.

CHAPTER ONE: JULIUS WAGNER-JAUREGG

Julius Wagner-Jauregg, born on March 7, 1857 to a prominent family in Wels, Upper Austria, was the son of Adolf Johann Wagner, a civil servant with a background in jurisprudence and politics (Whitrow, 1993). When his mother Ludovika succumbed to tuberculosis in 1867, his two sisters were resettled in a convent, while Julius and his brother Fritz remained at home. His father was transferred to Krems, a little town about 40 miles west of Vienna, and known for its apricot brandy, and then to Vienna in 1872. Later, when his father retired in 1883, he was made a nobleman and known as Ritter von Jauregg (derived from his mother's maiden name, Jauernigg), which was retained as a hyphenated name by his son even though such titles were generally eliminated after World War I.

After the move to Vienna, Julius continued his secondary education at the Schottengymnasium, a famous boys' school with origins as a Benedictine Abbey in 1807, which was popular with the nobility. Although there is a record that he graduated with honors, there is limited information about what he was like as a child and adolescent (his own memoirs begin in his university years). We do know that he suffered from typhoid during his childhood, and while in school is thought to have developed tuberculosis. As the family could not afford to send him to a sanatorium, he remained in school, sometimes stepping out to sit in a nearby park until his spells of coughing and bringing up bloody phlegm subsided. His health ultimately improved, and indeed he was very athletic most of his adult life, enjoying mountain trekking and doing calisthenics regularly.

Wagner-Jauregg began his studies at the prestigious University of Vienna in 1874. His father was said to have favored him going into philosophy, which took fewer years of training, but also recognized that medicine might be natural, recalling that he had a history of dissecting dead animals (Kleinert, 2022; Whitrow, 1993). Julius ultimately chose medicine, not long before enrolling. His memoirs and other materials provide little information as to how he came to this decision.

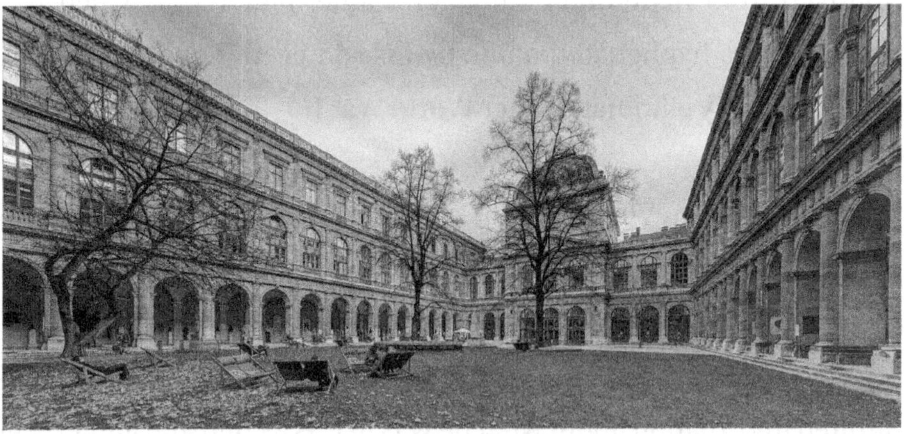

Figure 1-1: *A view of the main courtyard at the University of Vienna, which was built in 1877-1884, as seen in a 2015 photo.*

During his medical school years, Wagner-Jauregg did animal research in the laboratory of the pathologist Salomon Stricker, known for his histological studies of blood vessel walls, white blood cell movement into the site of infections, the cornea, and other subjects. Wagner-Jauregg developed skill in using laboratory animals in research, which was not widely done at the time, and published papers based on animal studies of nervous system regulation of heart rate and respiration. It was during his student years that he took some of the same courses as Sigmund Freud; the two became acquainted and began their long relationship.

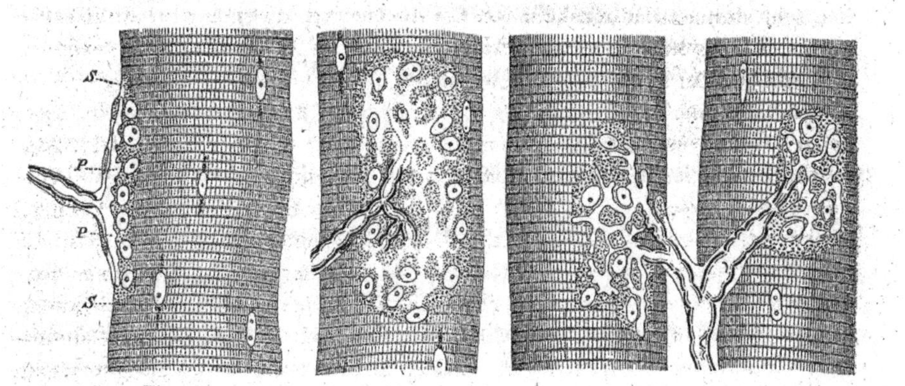

Figure 1-2: *This illustration shows a microscopic view of the attachment points (motor end plates) of the fibers of nerve cells to muscle tissue, as portrayed in Salomon Stricker's 1871 edited book* Manual of the Study of the Tissues of Man and Animals *(author's translation).*

After a year interrupted by military service, in which he was stationed in Vienna, Wagner-Jauregg graduated in 1880. He took an assistantship in Stricker's Institute of General and Experimental

Pathology, where a little later he and Freud briefly worked together. He had become interested in internal medicine while also working part-time in the university's clinics, and chose this as his career. His applications in 1882 to the two major programs in Vienna, however, were turned down. Uncertain what to do next, he was considering moving to Egypt when two professor acquaintances whom he saw at a coffeehouse mentioned that there was an open assistantship under Max von Leidesdorf at the First Psychiatric Clinic in Vienna's Asylum of Lower Austria. As Leidesdorf was a celebrated psychiatrist who was called upon to consult with royalty and was well-known for his studies of the relation of physical and mental disorders, this seemed an excellent opportunity. Though Wagner-Jauregg had had virtually no training in psychiatry, he applied the next day, and to his own surprise, was accepted. Armed with a hastily purchased textbook of psychiatry, he began his assistantship. By 1885 he was lecturing on neuropathology, and rose so rapidly that by 1887, when Leidesdorf was incapacitated by a heart attack, he was qualified in both psychiatry and neurology, and in effect began managing the clinic.

During these years, Wagner-Jauregg had become involved in research on two illnesses, hypothyroidism and the psychiatric and neurological consequences of syphilis infections. At Leidesdorf's request, he surgically removed the thyroid gland of cats, and observed their resulting sickness which was often fatal. He presented his data at a medical meeting, bringing along some of his unhappy feline patients by way of demonstration. He published his results in 1884, at about the same time as similar findings were made by the

German researcher, Moritz Schiff. These findings seemed to confirm the work of Emil Theodor Kocher, a Swiss surgeon who the year before had described clinical hypothyroidism in patients who had had thyroid tissue removed in the course of treating its various illnesses. Kocher went on to win the 1909 Nobel Prize for emphasizing aseptic techniques and greatly decreasing the mortality from thyroid surgery. Wagner-Jauregg did not pursue the thyroid studies at this time, but returned to them later (Chapter Three).

The second area of research which had started during Wagner-Jauregg's training was the study of dementia paralytica, or general paresis of the insane (see Appendix). This delayed consequence of syphilis which can appear many years after infection was responsible for up to one in five psychiatric hospitalizations before the development of modern treatments. Affected patients would develop personality changes, mood disorders, dementia, and disturbances of gait and coordination due to spinal tract involvement (tabes dorsalis), accompanied by tremors and seizures. While in Leidesdorf's clinic, Wagner-Jauregg had made the observation that some patients with mental disorders including dementia paralytica seemed to get better after contracting illnesses such as erysipelas and typhoid fever; he thought that this might be related to the fever they had produced.

By 1887, Wagner-Jauregg began to speculate whether purposely infecting patients with febrile illnesses such as erysipelas and malaria might benefit mental illnesses. He performed some preliminary studies with streptococci derived from erysipelas patients with little success, but later continued this approach with tuberculin, and then in 1917 with malaria, for which he was to win the Nobel Prize in 1927 (Chapter Three).

In 1889 Wagner-Jauregg moved to the University of Graz, well known for its scholarship but which also introduced him to the reality of limited resources and hardship in clinical psychiatric care away from the elite hospitals of Vienna. Before long he was also reminded of his earlier thyroid work. This area in southeastern Austria near the eastern portion of the Alps was known for its high rate of cretinism (a disorder of limited growth and impaired mental functioning) and goiter (a swelling of the neck due to an enlarged thyroid gland). While trekking in the mountains, Wagner-Jauregg saw many of these individuals, and for several months in 1892 began visiting some of these areas two days a week to study them. By the late 1890s it became clear that cretinism and one form of goiter were associated with thyroid malfunction due to inadequate dietary iodine, and he became a leader in the effort to require the addition of iodine to salt in Austrian areas prone to these disorders. Ultimately, such legislation was passed, though not until 1923. Opponents of this program got it rescinded in 1938, though it was re-introduced in 1944 after Wagner-Jauregg's death.

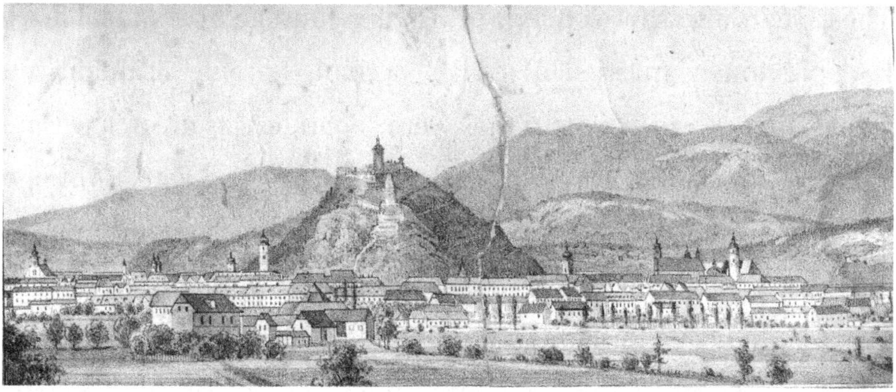

Figure 1-3: *Graz, seen in this 19th century drawing, is the second largest city in Austria (after Vienna) and has long been known as a center or learning, with four universities and four colleges. The University of Graz, which goes back to 1585, has had a remarkable group of faculty members over the years, including the 17th century astronomer Johannes Kepler; in the time period of this book, the Nobelist physiologist Otto Loewi taught there from 1909 to 1938, and the Nobelist physicist Erwin Schrödinger was chancellor in 1936. Nikola Tesla studied electricity at the city's University of Technology in 1875.*

In 1893 Wagner-Jauregg returned to Vienna when to his surprise he was offered the directorship of the First Psychiatric Clinic at the asylum in Vienna, along with a professorship at the University. During this period, Wagner-Jauregg also trained many outstanding students, including Constantin von Economo, who went on to make many contributions about the regulation of sleep and waking as well as the architecture of the cerebral cortex. Wagner-Jauregg became well known for having initiated medical education courses which were held four times a year, and attracted an international audience. He was also frequently asked to perform forensic evaluations, and became active in recommendations for revising laws regarding the criminally insane.

These years also saw a change in Wagner-Jauregg's personal life. He had previously married a Jewish woman, Balbine Frumkin, but things did not work out and they were separated, as divorce was not lawful at that point. He had then become involved with a younger woman, Anna Koch, who gave birth to their son Theodor. After his wife passed away, however, they were able to get married in 1899. His first marriage to Balbine Frumkin, however, was to become an issue four decades later when his political and racial views become more prominent (Chapter Four).

In 1902 Wagner-Jauregg moved to the Second Psychiatric Clinic at the General Hospital in Vienna, where he stayed until he retired in 1928. His work in those years was marked by his controversial treatments of mentally traumatized soldiers in World War I, and his Nobel Prize-winning development of malaria therapy for syphilis of the nervous system, as well as thyroid and ovarian therapy, and in some cases sterilization, for mental illness (Chapter Three).

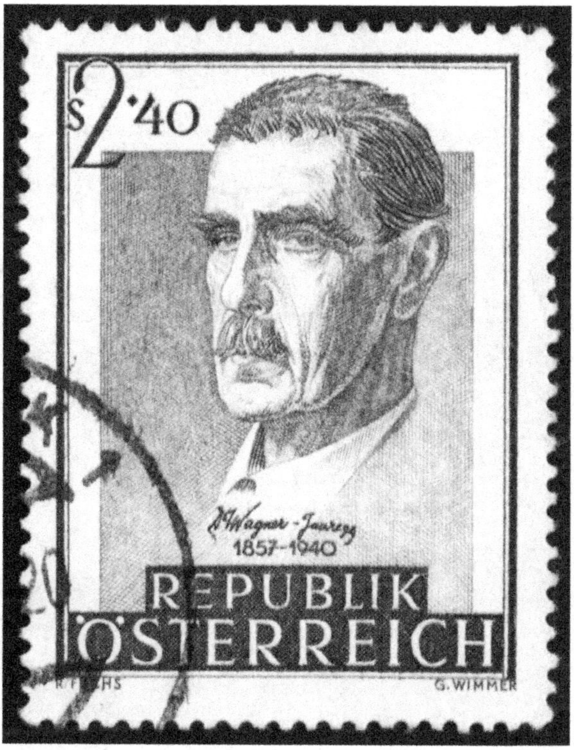

Figure 1-4: *Austrian postage stamp picturing Wagner-Jauregg in 1957, on the 100th anniversary of his birth.*

After retirement from the directorship of the clinic, Wagner-Jauregg remained very active, writing approximately 80 papers, among them the most comprehensive summary of his malaria treatment in 1931. His ideas about febrile therapy continued to evolve, and at age 82, a year before his death on September 27, 1940, he began to speculate on using chemical or physical means, rather than infection, to increase body temperature (Wagner-Jauregg, 1939). In his last years, he also began to be a supporter of what was known as racial hygiene, an advocate of sterilization of those considered to be genetically inferior, and a supporter of the Nazi party (Chapter Four).

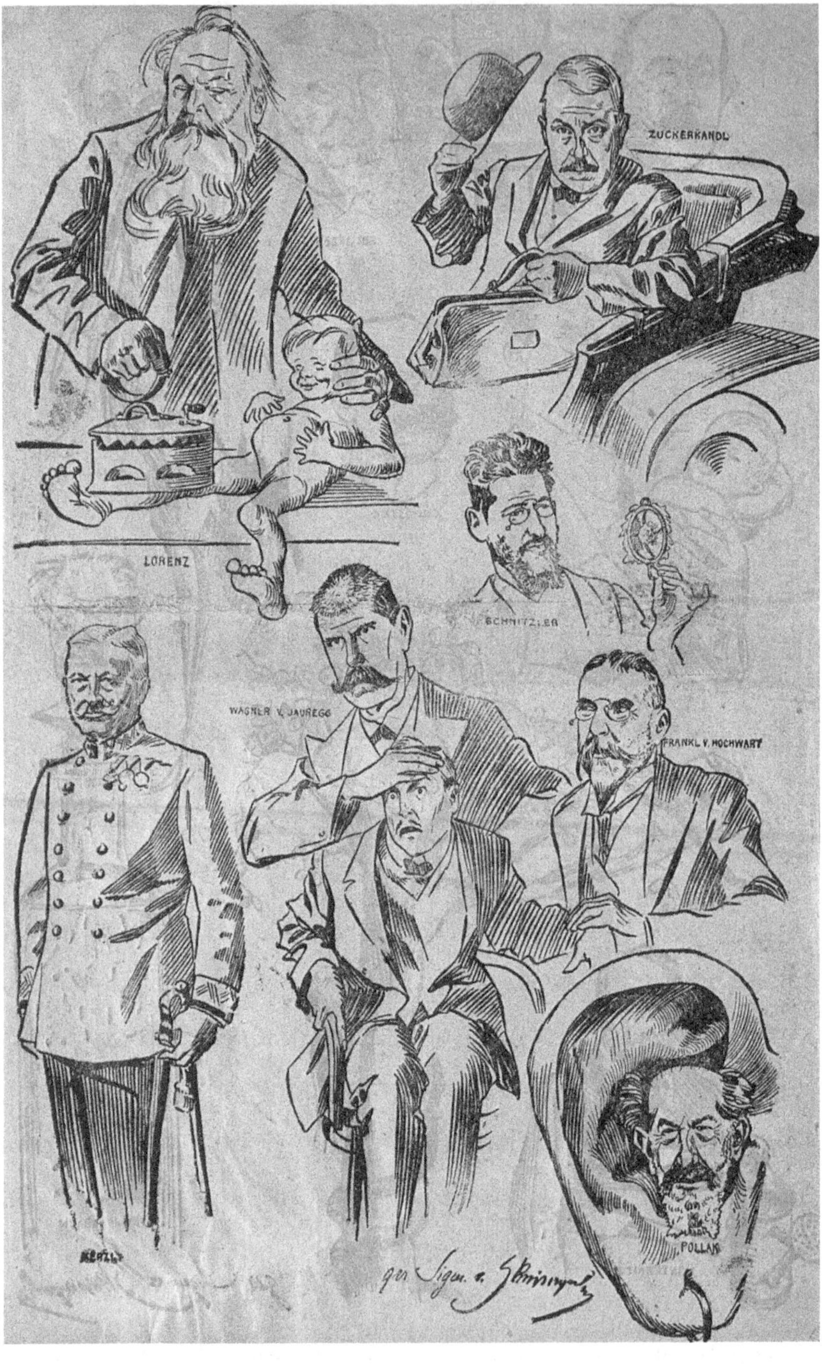

Figure 1-5: *This 1913 sketch of 'Seven Viennese Doctors' includes Wagner-Jauregg (center of second row, with his hand on patient's forehead).*

REFERENCES for CHAPTER ONE

Kleinert, R., in: Julius Wagner-Jauregg, in Whonamedit? A dictionary of medical eponyms. https://www.whonamedit.com/doctor.cfm/2753.html Accessed January 18, 2022.

Stricker, S. (ed): *Handbuch der Lehre von den Geweben des Menschen und der Thiere. (Manual of the study of the tissues of man and animals).* W. Englemann, Leipzig, 1871-1872.

Wagner-Jauregg, J. Derzeitige Behandlung der progressiven Paralyse. *Wien. Klin. Wochenschr.* **1939**, *52,* 1075–1078.

Whitrow, M.: Julius Wagner-Jauregg (1857-1940). J. Med. Biography 1: 137-143, 1993. https://journals.sagepub.com/doi/abs/10.1177/096777209300100302?journalCode=jmba

CHAPTER TWO: SIGMUND FREUD

Freud was born on May 6, 1856 in Freiberg, Moravia (then part of the Austrian Empire, now in the Czech Republic). His parents were both of Ashkenazi Jewish heritage, coming from Galicia, which now includes areas of Ukraine and Poland. His father, Jakob Freud, a twice-widowed wool merchant with two sons from a previous marriage, had limited success in his profession and at the time the family was renting rooms in a locksmith's house. Sigismund (later modified to Sigmund) was the first child of 20-year-old Amalia Freud, who later went on to give birth to seven other children, one of whom died in infancy. She referred to Sigmund as her 'golden Sigi', and he was to remember their relationship as something close to unconditional love, just as he tended to remember resentment and jealousy of his father. Many years later, in a period of introspection beginning in the mid-1890s, he was to dwell on these childhood memories which contributed to his creation of the concept of the Oedipus complex.

Jakob Freud's precarious finances necessitated the family to move in 1859, and after a brief stay in Leipzig, they settled in Vienna when Sigmund was age four, and there he stayed for most of the rest of his life. Vienna, a crowded and bustling capital, was a very different experience from the rural, forested Freiberg countryside. In some ways the Freuds experienced it as outsiders in a predominantly Catholic city, though they lived in the largely Jewish lower-class neighborhood of Leopoldstadt. Sigmund's awareness of the antisemitic atmosphere surrounding them may have led to compensating fantasies of being similar to Hannibal, the third century BC Semitic Carthaginian leader whose father had him pledge to wreak havoc on Rome (Crews, 2017). This and his family's modest situation may have led to his interest in other powerful figures such as Caesar, Alexander and Napoleon.

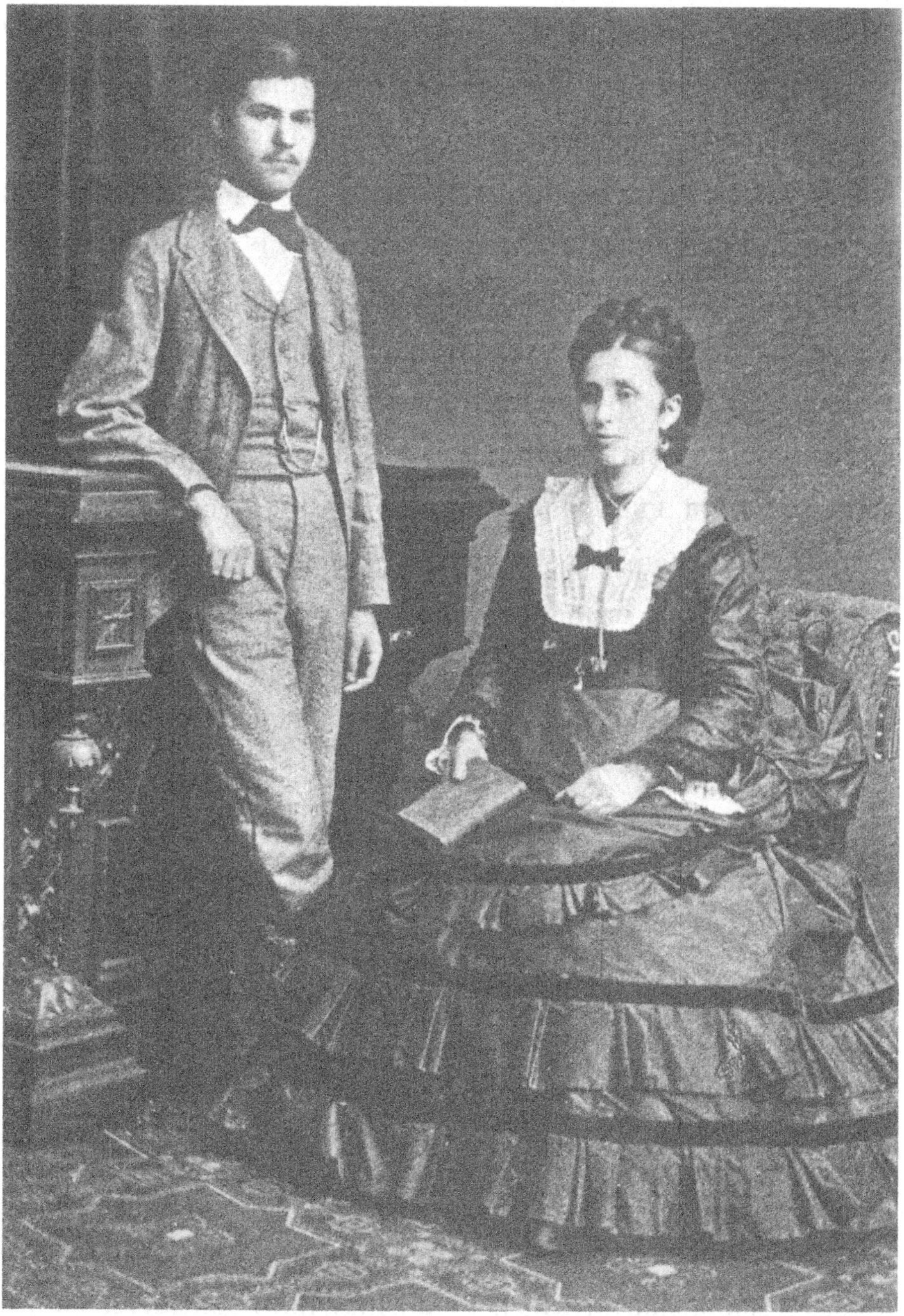

Figure 2-1: *Sigmund Freud, age 16, with his mother Amalia in 1872.*

Whatever misgivings Sigmund may have had about his community and station, he prospered in school, and by the time he graduated from secondary school with honors he spoke five languages. As an adolescent, he had been drawn to becoming a lawyer and entering politics. By the time he reached the University of Vienna in 1873 at the early age of 17, he was inclined toward science and medicine, according to some because he had been particularly moved by the writings of Goethe about nature. Even after switching to medicine, he continued to pursue other interests including philosophy and zoology. At one point he went to Trieste for a month to study the reproductive systems of eels under his zoology professor Carl Claus. He began working in the laboratory of Ernst von Brücke, a well-known physiologist/physician, and a leader in the notion that the methods of natural science could be used to elucidate how humans think and behave. Freud's investigations in Brücke's Institute of Physiology led him into many areas, including the anatomy of the eye, and what later came to be termed the cytoskeleton (internal structure) of nerve cells (Frixione, 2003). By the time Freud graduated, he had published six papers on various aspects of neuroanatomy, including the structure of the spinal cord as seen in fish, and the embryology of the nervous system. It was also in Brücke's laboratories that he met Joseph Breuer, a private practitioner some 14 years his senior, with a background in physiology and a continued interest in research. They were to form a close relationship in which Freud may have considered him a father figure, visiting frequently at his home and years later naming his first daughter after Breuer's wife. As we will see later, Breuer was also to play an important role in Freud's evolving view of hysteria.

In 1879 Freud began the required year's military service, which apparently did not keep him very busy, as he found time to translate into German a number of essays by the English philosopher John Stuart Mills. Freud later graduated in 1881. He had entered earlier, and graduated later, than Wagner-Jauregg, apparently because his other interests led him on a more circuitous course to medicine.

In 1882, as we mentioned earlier, Freud and Wagner-Jauregg, who both became involved in neuropathology work at Stricker's institute, decided to devote their careers to internal medicine. They both applied for the same jobs at the two university programs, and were turned down. As we described earlier, Jauregg, casting about for work, stumbled upon a position in psychiatry at a prestigious university-affiliated clinic located in the Asylum in Vienna. Freud, who was also in financial straits, was advised by his mentor Brücke to leave academics, and moved to the General Hospital, were he worked in various capacities, but particularly in the university's Second Psychiatric Clinic.

The clinic director, Theodor Meynert, was a psychiatrist and brain anatomist who had made substantial advances in understanding the structure of the cerebral cortex, and devoted himself to grounding psychiatry in brain anatomy. He believed that abnormal brain development increased the likelihood of having mental illness, and that psychoses, which he saw as disturbances in the relation of the cortex to deeper centers, were potentially reversible. Over the years, his list of remarkable students was also to include Sergei Korsakoff and Carl Wernicke, who were to later describe a psychotic state due to thiamine deficiency, and Auguste Forel, who recognized that neurons were the basic functional units in the nervous system.

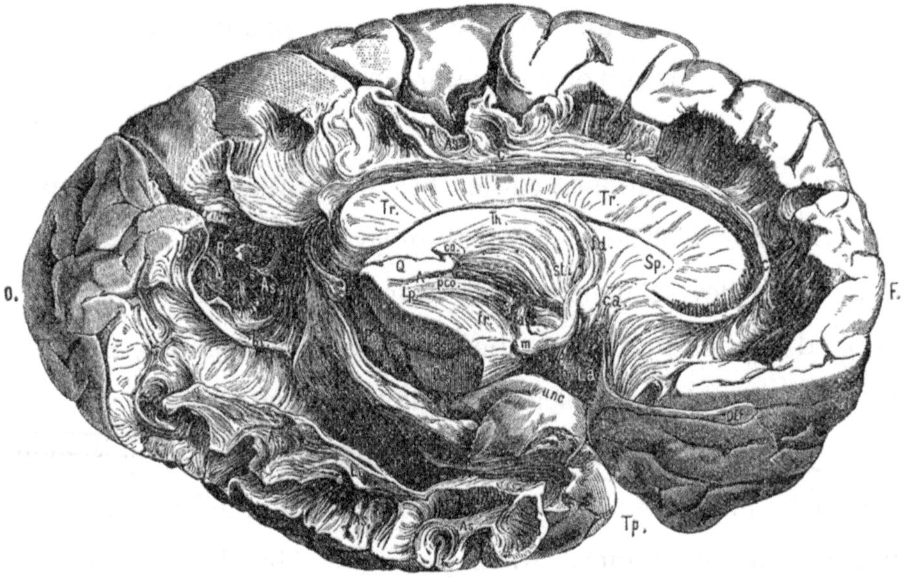

Figure 2-2: *Illustration of brain anatomy taken from Meynert's 1885 book,* A Clinical Treatise on Diseases of the Forebrain Based Upon a Study of its Structure, Functions and Nutrition.

Freud worked in a number of areas in those years. His clinical assessments of aphasic patients laid the foundation for a book on the topic he was to publish some time later in 1891; this and his assignment at an asylum sparked his enthusiasm for clinical care. During this period, he also became involved in studies of cocaine, which though partially successful in that he found some benefits related to eye surgery, led to the addiction of a colleague he was trying to help, and overall harmed his reputation. He continued to work part-time in Stricker's laboratory with Wagner-Jauregg, and in 1884 the two of them brokered peace between two eye surgeons who both claimed to have been the first to take advantage of the analgesic effects of cocaine. Freud himself appeared to use cocaine in the years 1884-1887. Some believe that this may have persisted as late as 1896, with encouragement for taking it for migraine relief from his colleague Wilhelm Fleiss ,who will appear later in this chapter (Goleman, 1985).

In 1885, Freud and Wagner-Jauregg both successfully applied for what was known as 'Habilitation', the awarding of the unpaid status of *Dozentur*, which meant that they could lecture on neuropathology at the University of Vienna. Freud, who was doing less well financially than Wagner-Jauregg, also requested support from the university, and received a travel grant to study in Paris under Jean-Martin Charcot. Though it was possible for him to get a six-month leave from the General Hospital, he resigned his position there (Whitrow, 1990).

Freud was drawn to Charcot's work with hysteria, sometimes then described as 'ungovernable emotional excess' in which patients (initially mostly women) would develop paralyses, difficulty speaking, bizarre facial expressions, tics and other symptoms for which no physiological cause could be found. Although Charcot's findings have been challenged over the years, he seemed to be showing that these mysterious paralyses could be relieved by hypnotic suggestion, and that conversely he could use hypnosis to induce such symptoms in non-patients. The implication seemed to be that there were levels of mental functioning which occurred outside of a person's conscious awareness, a notion that was a foundation of Freud's later work.

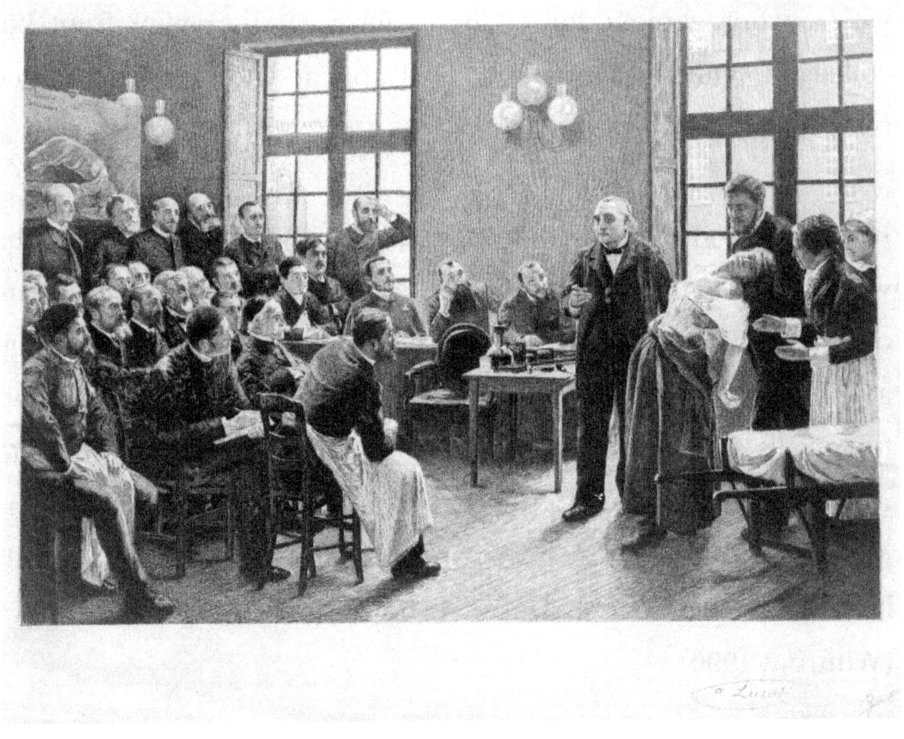

Figure 2-3: *Jean-Martin Charcot, a founder of modern neurology, at the Salpêtrière Hospital. Built in the sixteenth century for the manufacture of guns, it became a hospital in the seventeenth century and in Charcot's hands grew into one of the leading neurological centers of its day. He had a longstanding history of studying illnesses such as Parkinson's disease, multiple sclerosis and amyotrophic lateral sclerosis ('Lou Gehrig's disease'), and became very interested in hysteria. He believed that there was often a history of trauma, including sexual experiences, some years before Freud did, and that hypnosis and hysteria produced similar*

mental states (Bogousslavsky, 2011). This 1888 etching depicts Charcot demonstrating his hypnotic techniques in his clinic, in a manner which has sometimes been described as 'spectacular, even theatrical' (Schneck,1961).

After studying with Charcot for about five months, Freud's return to Vienna in 1886 led to two major changes in his life. He married Martha Bernays, with whom he had had a relationship for the last four years, and ultimately went on to have six children. At Breuer's urging, he also established a private office devoted to what he termed 'nervous disorders'. He was influenced no doubt by Breuer's success in the role of private physician/scientist, as well as his offer to refer him patients. Freud was to go on to maintain his practice until 1938.

Breuer, whose history included elucidating the role of the inner ear in the sense of balance, and co-discovering a respiratory reflex (the Hering-Breuer reflex), had an excellent background in neuroanatomy. Freud, however, was taken with another aspect of his interests, stemming from his treatment of a 21 year old patient named Bertha Pappenheim ('Anna O'). Pappenheim, about whom Freud had first learned in 1882, and never met, had developed a variety of symptoms upon her father's terminal illness with tuberculosis. She suffered from mysterious paralyses, loss of sensation, a nervous cough, hallucinations, and a reluctance to eat. Breuer, following her inclinations, initially allowed her to invent fantasy tales, after which she seemed to feel better, in a process she referred to as 'chimney sweeping'. He later used daily hypnosis, which he approached from a somewhat different direction than Charcot, considering it a way of finding the causes of hysteria. Later, he found that he did not need to induce hypnosis himself, and instead allowed her to slip into a kind of self-hypnotic state. While in this condition she was able to recover the memory of a traumatic event. As she did so, her symptoms became more intense, but then afterwards seemed to improve. In one famous example, Pappenheim, who was having difficulty drinking, recalled her feelings when she saw a dog lick water from a woman's glass; once having relived this experience, she was better able to take fluids.

Pappenheim came to think of her treatment, in her words, as the 'talking cure'. Looking back, the cure may not have been as complete as might have been hoped. By the end of her treatment in 1882 her symptoms were severe, and Breuer, who was giving her morphine for trigeminal nerve (facial) pain, had her hospitalized. Some modern critics later suggested that although Freud lauded the benefits of Breuer's techniques, he 'always knew that the treatment of Bertha Pappenheim...had not been an unmitigated success' (Borch-Jacobsen and Shamdasani, 2012). Ultimately she got better, and went on to a career of helping orphans and single mothers, becoming well known as an advocate for the rights of women.

Despite the complex outcome of Bertha Pappenheim, the idea of catharsis, that the movement of a memory from the unconscious to conscious expression was curative, became central to Freud's early thinking. Some years later he came to believe that hypnosis was unreliable, and that insight into the unconscious could come from 'free association' allowing the patient to relax and say whatever came to mind. Nonetheless, the idea of the unconscious mind, and the uses of hypnosis which he first advocated, were unpopular, and were not convincing to either his erstwhile teacher Theodor Meynert nor to Wagner-Jauregg.

Meynert seemed particularly incensed with Freud's notion of male hysteria. This conflict had the interesting twist that the mentor himself may have been concealing hysteric-like symptoms and had a rapprochement with Freud in Meynert's last years (Faucher, 1996). Freud's recognition may also have been limited by his early focus on neuroses, which, as opposed to psychoses, were initially not considered part of mainstream psychiatry. Moreover, in those years middle-class Viennese society honored, at least on the surface, a form of rigid morality that in some ways may have surpassed that of their Victorian counterparts in Britain (Shaw, 2021). Thus views which emphasized the sexual drives were seen as suspect; this may have been even more so in the psychiatric community, which was growing more aware of the ravages of syphilis, which was seen as resulting from excessive sexual activity (see Appendix). A subtler barrier to acceptance may have been a reaction to Freud and Breuer's Jewish backgrounds, though the degree to which antisemitism played a role in these early professional years has been argued back and forth over time (see Appendix).

In 1895 Freud and Breuer published their book *Studies in Hysteria,* which if anything polarized opinions even more. One newspaper review disparagingly called it 'the kind of psychology used by poets' (von Bergner, 1895), while the English physician and social reformer Havelock Ellis and the Swiss psychiatrist Eugen Bleuler praised it. (The latter, however, remained unconvinced that the patients' improvement was not due to suggestion.) Most agreed, however, that *Studies in Hysteria* made Freud's name much more widely known both locally and abroad. It also marked the end of a declining relationship with Breuer, who was not prepared to accept Freud's belief that sexuality lay at the heart of most neuroses. Freud felt resentful at what he considered to be a failure in supporting his work. Their breakup was seemingly complete, though Freud felt touched to learn after Breuer's death much later in 1925 that he had sympathetically been keeping track of Freud's work over the years (DesGroseillers, 1999).

By 1896, Freud was referring to his techniques as psychoanalysis. As the years passed, his thinking continued to evolve. He differed from Charcot and Breuer in the almost exclusive emphasis on the role of sexual memories in the development of female hysteria. He originally formulated the notion of 'seduction theory', suggesting that childhood sexual trauma which was held in the unconscious ('repressed') was the keystone to the development of neuroses. He later came to think that fantasies of such trauma also might be responsible, but whether real or imagined, the contribution to neuroses occurred if they became repressed.

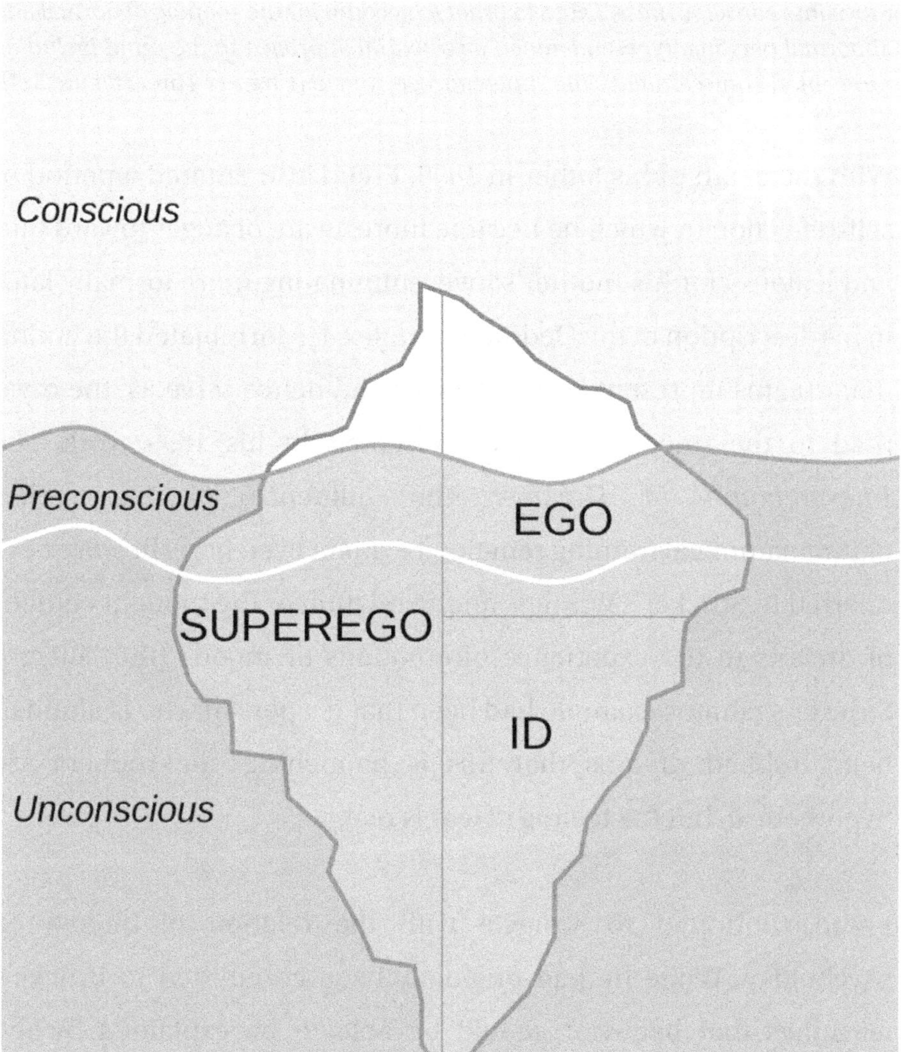

Figure 2-4: *Freud's 'topographic' conception of the mind, with roots in his 1895* Project for a Scientific Psychology, *suggested that the conscious mind is only one of three components, the top layer of what is sometimes pictured as an iceberg. Conscious processes are capable of recognizing the difference between reality and our inner thoughts, considering the future, and responding to society's needs. Beneath is the unconscious, home of basic drives and repressed memories. Between them is the preconscious, containing a mixture of logical thought and irrational fantasies of which we are not immediately aware, but which can readily*

move into consciousness. Later, in order to account for the shaping of normal and abnormal personality, Freud added a structural approach to the mind including three interacting elements, the superego, ego, and id (Chapter Three; Figure 3-3).

With the death of his father in 1896, Freud also entered a period of self-reflection in which he became more aware of anger toward him and jealousy for his mother's love, culminating more formally later in his description of the Oedipus complex. He formulated the notion that dreams represent hidden wishes and hence serve as 'the royal road to the unconscious', as presented in his 1899 work *The Interpretation of Dreams.* The influence of his earlier neuroanatomical training remained evident even here, however. He referred to Stricker's writings on the relation of the thought content of dreams to the experience of emotions or moods (the 'affect'). Stricker's famous example had been that if a person who is afraid of being robbed dreams that this is happening, the robbers are hypothetical, but the feeling of fear is real

Freud continued to struggle with the relation of biology to psychology. While he had originally been committed to Brücke's teachings that behavior should be able to be explained by the principles of biology, his observations of his patients' actions suggested that they followed very different kinds of laws (Barondes, 1990). He described the history of these struggles in 1895 in *Project for a Scientific Psychology,* which was not published until after his death. This particular work was derived from letters to Wilhelm Fleiss, a Berlin otolaryngologist to whom Freud had been introduced by Breuer in 1887. Fleiss held a number of ideas such as the similarity of nasal and genital tissues, and that disorders of the latter could be treated by surgery on the former. He also believed in a kind of biorhythmic study based on the notion of periodicities in males and females of 23 and 28 days duration, which he believed could predict a great deal of human behavior. One of his more disastrous predictions, incidentally, was that Freud would die at age 51, which turned out to be off by some three decades. He also advocated the use of nasal cocaine for relieving a variety of disorders.

Although Fleiss' notions about the nasal mucosa and biorhythms have since been repudiated, he served as a confident with whom Freud could share his personal thoughts, a friendly listener to Freud's ideas during a time in his career at which few were attentive (Goleman, 1985). Some believe that he might have contributed to Freud's growing concept of infantile sexuality (Sulloway, 1979). Their friendship was to deteriorate and then end a few years later after Fleiss accused Freud of inappropriately borrowing his ideas in 1900. It is possible that the arc of the relationship was similar to the one Freud had had with Breuer: an initial enthusiasm or even idealization of the other's beliefs, followed by disillusion, resentful feelings of not being supported, and breakup (Goleman, 1885). One interpretation of Freud's later unhappy relations with some of his students such as Carl Jung and Sandor Ferenczi has been that these, too, followed a similar pattern.

In the next few years Freud also began to explore a number of other areas. He asserted, for instance, that common occurrences such as slips of the tongue, forgetting names, or telling jokes might provide clues to unconscious conflicts of more recent vintage, not necessarily going back to infancy (*The Psychopathology of Everyday Life, 1901; Jokes and their Relation to the Unconscious, 1905).* He expanded his thoughts about dream interpretation, and he wrote, among other things, about creativity, narcissism, obsessional neurosis, psychopathic characters in drama, and taboos among indigenous peoples. (A detailed description of the development of his thinking is found in Whitebook, 2017).

While expanding the range of psychoanalytic thought, Freud was also aware of the importance of having platforms from which to present his ideas. He realized that they would likely be given more weight coming from a professor, and tried to overcome his status as an outsider by obtaining a university position. In 1899 his efforts were made more difficult by a letter for the promotion board by Wagner-Jauregg, noting Freud's background in neuropathology and saying that 'he has never really worked in psychiatry' (Whitrow, 1990). In 1902 he finally became 'Professor extraordinarius', a lesser posting for a professor without a chair, usually in a marginal area of study. Interestingly, one story (Philips, 2014) has it that he obtained this position only after an ex-patient, the Baroness Marie Ferstel, used the gift of a painting to influence a government official's decision. (We will see later in Chapter Four that Freud's prestigious patients once again came to his rescue when he was in a difficult situation with the Gestapo.) His new title, however, made it easier for Freud to continue his lectures at the university.

In 1919 Freud finally became 'Professor ordinarius', or professor with a chair and who is involved in a more traditional area of study, but even then this was largely a titular rank (Whitrow, 1990). This, too, had been difficult to achieve, partially due to a rather tepid endorsement by Wager-Jauregg, who noted that Freud's notions were likely to be disproven but were based on original observations which should be appreciated.

Overall, Freud's slow pathway in academics was in marked contrast to that of Wagner-Jauregg, who had always held traditional university ranks and had been a full Professor of Psychiatry since 1893. In passing, it should be mentioned that their paths toward a Nobel Prize differed as well. Wagner-Jauregg was nominated, and received, the Nobel in 1927. Freud, in contrast, was nominated 13 times (12 in medicine and once in literature) between 1915 and 1938, but he never won. It is said that even Einstein, perhaps concerned about his radical views, failed to support him.

A few months after Freud's first professorship in 1902, he began to hold regular Wednesday evening gatherings in his home, and over time attracted a remarkable group of colleagues such as Alfred Adler and Otto Rank. By 1908 the group grew into the more formal Vienna Psychoanalytic Society, of which Freud was the first president. The energy of the movement attracted physicians from abroad. Among these were Ernest Jones, a London neurologist, and Carl Jung, a psychiatrist at the University of Zurich who had studied the galvanic skin response and word association tests, and who had a growing interest in unconscious processes. In 1910 the International Psychoanalytic Society was formed, led, at Freud's suggestion, by Jung. Though its activities were filled with intellectual disagreements, personal strife, and defections (among these, a split with Alfred Adler in 1911 and Jung in 1913), it represented a growing movement and major force in psychiatric thought.

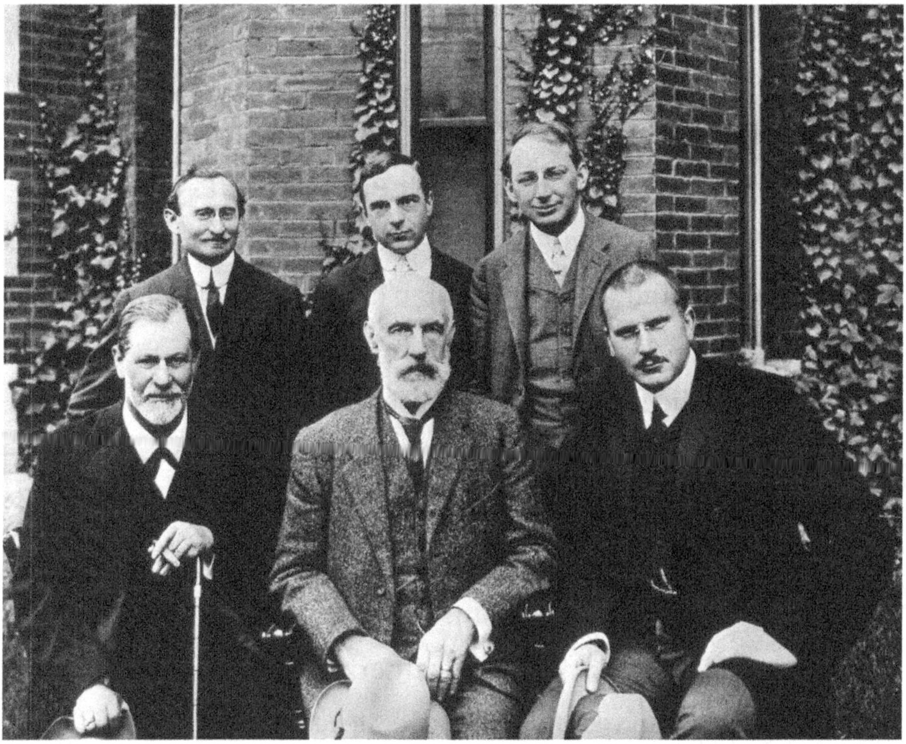

Figure 2-5: *Freud and some of his followers, 1909.* Front row (left to right): *Freud, Stanley Hall, Carl Jung.* Back row: *Abraham Arden Brill, Ernest Jones and Sándor Ferenczi.*

By this point Freud was in his late 50s, the founder of an important new field. It was in in this period that World War I broke out. The wartime years were to have profound effects on his thinking, which expanded to considerations of society and aggressiveness from the psychoanalytic viewpoint. The postwar years began with a difficult time in which Freud was called on to pass judgment on Wagner-Jauregg's work (Chapter Three), and continued into the 1920s, when he developed a 'structural' view of the mind involving the interplay of the ego, id, and superego (*Freud,* 1923). In the 1930s, he began to be targeted by the rising Nazi party which instigated burnings of his books. After the German annexation of Austria in 1938 he was persecuted by the Gestapo; he ultimately fled to London, where he passed away on September 23, 1939 (Chapter Four). His ashes were placed in a third century BC Greek urn, a gift from his ever-loyal patient, Princess Marie Bonaparte, and remain in London.

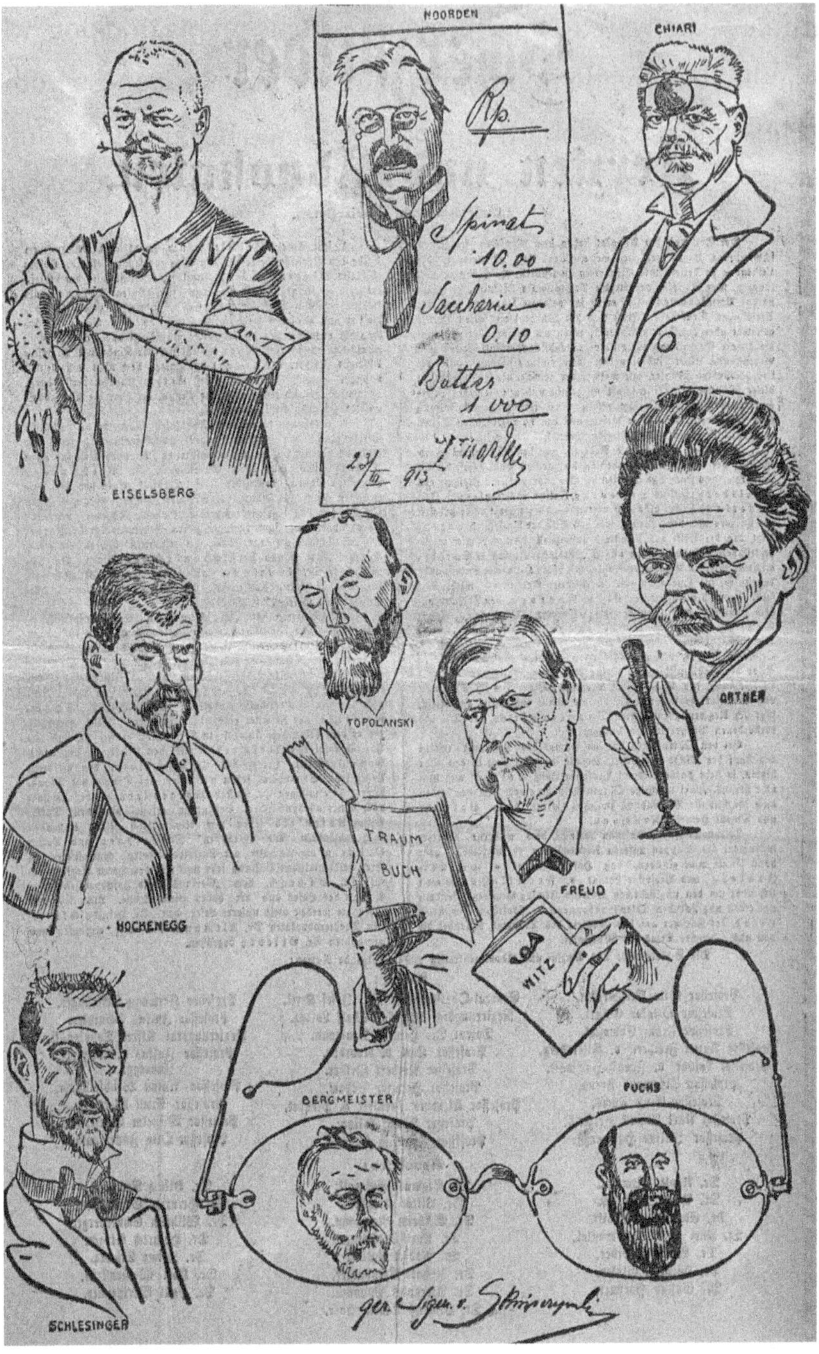

Figure 2-6: *This 1913 sketch of 'Ten Viennese Doctors' shows Freud, the third figure from the left in the second row, reading a book.*

REFERENCES for CHAPTER TWO

Barondes, S.H.: The biological approach to psychiatry: history and prospects. J. Neurosci. 10: 1707-1710, 1990. https://www.jneurosci.org/content/jneuro/10/6/1707.full.pdf

Borch-Jacobsen, Mikkel; Shamdasani, Sonu: *The Freud Files: An Inquiry into the History of Psychoanalysis.* Cambridge: Cambridge University Press. pp. 56, 107, 166 (2012) ISBN 978-0-521-72978-9.

Bogousslavsky, J.: Hysteria after Charcot: back to the future. Front. Neurol. Neurosci. 29: 137-161, 2011. https://pubmed.ncbi.nlm.nih.gov/20938153/

Crews, F.: *Freud: the Making of an Illusion,* 2017, p. 11.

DesGroseillers, R.A.: Joseph Breuer, in Freudfile.org. https://www.freudfile.org/breuer.html (Accessed February 26, 2022).

Fancher, R., E.: *Pioneers of Psychology (3rd eds).* Norton and Company Inc., London/New York, 1996.

Freud, S.: *The Interpretation of Dreams.* Basic Books, 2010 (Original text 1899).

Freud, S.: *The Psychopathology of Everyday Life.* Andesite Press, 2015 edition. (Original text 1901).

Freud, S.: *The Ego and the Id.* W.W. Norton & Co., 1990 edition. (Original text 1923).

Freud, S., & Bonaparte, M., Freud, A., & Kris, E. (Eds.). (1954). *Project for a scientific psychology* (E. Mosbacher & J. Strachey, Trans.). In S. Freud & M. Bonaparte, A. Freud, E. Kris (Eds.) & E. Mosbacher, J. Strachey (Trans.),: *The origins of psycho-analysis: Letters to Wilhelm Fliess, drafts and notes: 1887-1902* (pp. 347–445). Basic Books. https://doi.org/10.1037/11538-013

Freud, S. and J. Breuer: *Studies in hysteria,* Penguin Classics, 2004. (Original text published in 1895).

Frixione, E.: Sigmund Freud's contribution to the history of the neuronal cytoskeleton. J. Hist. Neurosci. 12: 12-24, 2003. https://pubmed.ncbi.nlm.nih.gov/12785109/

Goleman, D.: New insights into Freud. New York Times Magazine, March 17, 1985. https://www.nytimes.com/1985/03/17/magazine/new-insights-into-freud.html (Accessed February 26, 2022).

Meynert, T.: Psychiatry. A Clinical Treatise on Diseases of the Forebrain Based Upon a Study of its Structure, Functions and Nutrition, Part 1. The Anatomy, Physiology, and Chemistry of the Brain. Translated by B. Sachs. New York, G.P. Putnams' Sons, 1885. Reprinted in: Neurosciences, Vol. 15, No. 4, July 2006: pp. 1–62 Cerebral White Matter — Historical Evolution of Facts and Notions Concerning the Organization of the Fiber Pathways of the Brain. Journal of the History of the Neurosciences, 16:237–267, 2007

Phillips, Adam: *Becoming Freud:* Yale University Press, 2014 p. 139.'

Schneck, J.M.: Jean-Martin Charcot and the history of experimental hypnosis. J. History of Medicine and Allied Sciences. 16: 297-305, 1961.
https://www.jstor.org/stable/24620683

Sulloway, F.J.: *Freud, Biologist of the Mind.* Basic Books, 1979.

Von Bergner, A.: Neue Freie Presse, December 2, 1895.

Whitebook,J.: *Freud, an intellectual biography.* Cambridge University Press, 2017.

Whitrow, M.: Freud and Wagner-Jauregg: A historiographical study. Psychiatric Bulletin 14: 356-358, 1990.

CHAPTER THREE: WORLD WAR I AND ITS AFTERMATH—MELANCHOLY AND MALARIA

Effect on Freud's thinking

At the outbreak of World War I in 1914, Freud, like many in the Austria-Hungary, was generally enthusiastic, and he commented that for the first time in years, it made him feel very much an Austrian. His only hesitation was that it was difficult for him to think of England as being on the other side, and he was quick to let his English follower Ernest Jones know that he was not viewed as an enemy. His three sons, though initially rejected or exempted from service, ultimately volunteered for service.

Later, Freud began to recognize the extent of the wholesale destruction, and that it was likely to last a long time. As a son-in-law returned home wounded in 1916 and a nephew was killed in 1917, he became weary and discouraged. At a political level it was especially hard to see the breakdown of the *Pax Britannica*, which had upheld Western values and provided relative stability for decades (Freud Library, 1985). Gone was the Enlightenment ideal of a civilized Europe in which art and philosophy could peacefully flourish.

Freud's disillusion with the war affected his thinking in at least two important ways. First, he began to find it even harder to retain his commitment to finding physiologic causes of behavior (Gay, 1995). Even his initial depiction of the mind being comprised of conscious, unconscious and preconscious components (the 'topographical model') had retained some biological underpinnings consistent with this history. Now, rather than focusing primarily on the role of the sexual impulse and its repression as the origin of neuroses, he came to believe that much of human behavior could be explained by the opposition of two powerful forces: 'Eros', the drive for love, and 'Thanatos', the predilection for aggression and violence. In his *Thoughts for the Times on War and Death* (Freud, 1916), written when the war had been progressing for only about six months, he expressed this view, along with the disappointment in society's ability to provide adequate safeguards.

Freud began to explore the implications of loss and depressed mood in his 1917 book *Mourning and Melancholia.* He also began to recognize man as a social animal. Instead of focusing on the individual and the relationship to parents, he saw the role the role of society in shaping morals and helping keep aggression under control. In his terms, this suggested that the community plays a role in the development of the superego (see Figure 3-3). One implication of these thoughts was emphasizing the importance of providing readily available treatment for mental illness, and as time went on the second generation of psychoanalysts began to provide free community-based clinics (Danto, 2016).

In 1930 Freud published *Civilization and its Discontents.* In it, he pictured civilization as a force that replays upon the cultural stage the same conflicts which are found inside the individual psyche—the repression of the drives for sexual and aggressive expression, which he considered immutable. Phrased differently, he began to take the view that human unhappiness results not only because of repressed sexuality, but also because of the restraints which society places on very fundamental aggressive and destructive instincts (Shaw, 2021). He also had the sobering realization that sometimes this does not work, and that collectively, large bodies of people can overwhelm the moral restraints of the individual and actually unleash the horrors of war (Coblence, 2022). He began to realize that depending on the circumstance, society's influence could either help control or alternatively breed aggression (Shaw, 2021). As we will see later in this chapter, this view led him to consider a new way of viewing the source of shell shock in soldiers.

Wagner-Jauregg and the treatment of shell shock

A brief history of shell shock:

Psychiatric reactions to trauma have been recorded going back to ancient Sumer in the second millennium BC. In the epic of Gilgamesh, the titular hero undergoes grief at the death of his companion Enkidu, then becomes depressed, suffers recurring dreams of the trauma, and focuses on his own mortality. As described in the companion book *Trial by Fire* (Mendelson, 2021), the Bible describes soldiers whose emotional reaction caused them to be sent home (Deuteronomy 20: 1-9), and in the fifth century BC, the Greek historian Herodotus reported that some soldiers appeared to become blind though not physically injured.

As agonizing as these wars in antiquity must have been, they were surpassed by the sheer volume of killing in World War I. The battle of the Somme, for instance, resulted in over one million casualties with 300,000 fatalities (O'Neill, 2022).

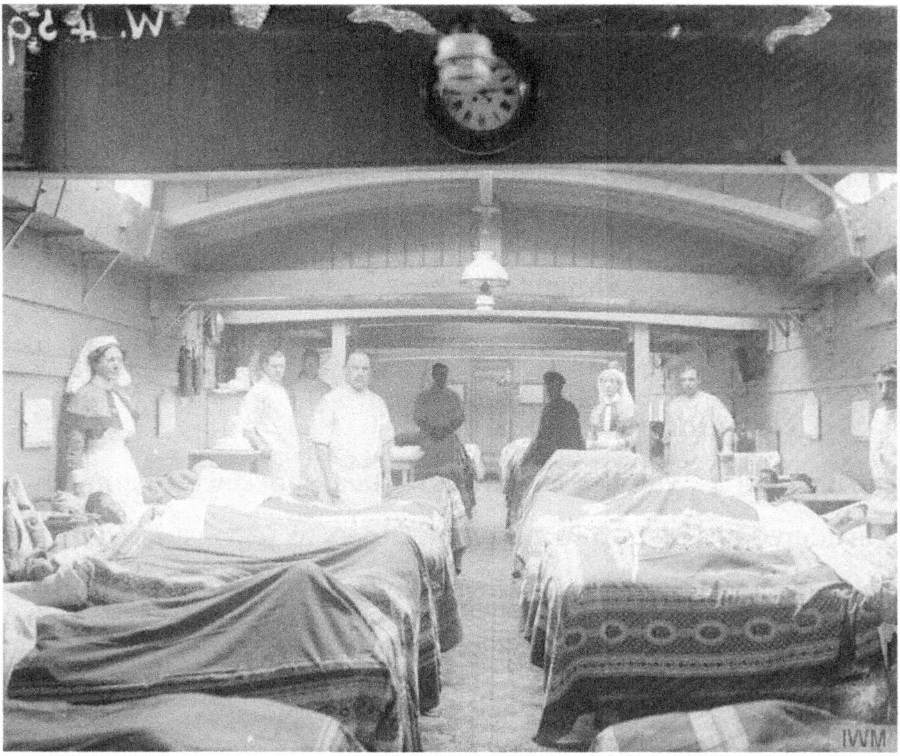

Figure 3-1: *The 'industrial' scale of violence in World War I presented an unprecedented challenge for caring for the wounded. Pictured here is a barge reconfigured by the British into a mobile hospital, as used in the canals of France and Flanders.*

By some estimates, 40 percent of casualties during the war suffered from the condition which came to be known as shell shock or war neurosis, and up to 80 percent were not able to return to battle (BBC, 2004). Many developed severe anxiety and depression, decreased appetite, palpitations, apparent blindness, paralyses or loss of speech, insomnia and nightmares. In more modern times there has been growing recognition that this kind of reaction can occur from non-military traumas as well and that the manifestations may not necessarily involve dramatic symptoms such as blindness. It is currently described as involving disturbances in cognition, mood and arousal, and including difficulties with impulsive acts and anger. It has been referred to in the nomenclature of the American Psychiatric Association as Post-Traumatic Stress Disorder since 1980. (For a more detailed description of the condition in modern terms, please see Friedman, 2021.)

The military response:

During World War I, soldiers with shell shock were sometimes considered deserters, and executed. Others were considered ill, and hospitals in all the participating countries were flooded with such patients. As the war progressed, there was also a movement toward retaining the soldiers for treatment in forward centers within the sound of the guns (Crocq, 2000).

A number of therapies were developed, and to some degree varied by country (Scharf, 2022). The French neurosurgeon Clovis Vincent developed the technique of 'torpedoing', in which 'persuasion' was paired with electric shocks, though this was abandoned after his patients rebelled against what they perceived as torture (Bogousslavsky, 2011). One patient, indeed, struck him, leading to a well-publicized trial. In Germany, hypnosis was used in some medical centers. Others viewed the diagnosis of shell shock with suspicion, likening it to malingering after industrial accidents. Some viewed it as being a form of hysteria (Blakemore, 2019). The soldiers were often considered unpatriotic or lazy, and treated with harsh disciplinary measures.

In Austria, the approach varied in different areas. In Graz, emphasis was placed on rest, nutrition, warm baths, and soothing activities. In Vienna, where Wagner-Jauregg practiced, electrical treatments were often employed. It was thought that shell shock was usually manifest in 'degenerates' and shirkers. Treatments, then, took on a punitive quality, with a goal being to differentiate those with true symptoms from those who were malingering. Methods varied, but could include applying electrodes to the seemingly afflicted area (for instance, to the throat of a soldier who had lost speech), and progress to shocks to sensitive areas such as the genitals. These could be accompanied by military drill, shaming or solitary confinement. One of the most extreme--and widely used-- methods was designed by the German psychiatrist Fritz Kaufmann, who advocated treatment in even a single session which emphasized military authority and suggestion techniques, accompanied by unrelenting shocks (Kaufmann, 1916). The unfortunate patient, it was thought, would have little choice but to flee back to the battleground.

Some have suggested that electrical therapy was particularly suited to the situation of the Austria-Hungarian Empire, which included troops from a variety of regions speaking a number of different languages. The reasoning was that, unlike hypnosis, minimal verbal communication was involved in electrical treatment (Scharf, 2022).

Whether or not this was the case, it is clear that the emphasis was on discipline if not actual punishment.

Wagner-Jauregg and shell shock:

When war broke out, Wagner-Jauregg was 57 and had long since completed his military obligation in his student days. Nonetheless, he was affected in that many of the patients in his hospital were soldiers with head injuries or shell shock, and sometimes unable to speak (Kleinert, 2022). He published extensively about shell shock based on his experience with these patients, and became a leading proponent of an aggressive form of electrical therapy. Ultimately knowledge about this method became more widespread, and reports that it was not very effective in returning troops to battle led to public resistance (Scharf, 2022).

Shortly after the end of the war, an Austrian commission was established in December 1918 to determine whether dereliction of duty had contributed to the defeat. Among the complaints it received was one from an officer who felt he had been mistreated by Wagner-Jauregg. A Lieutenant Kauders told the commission that he had suffered a head injury in battle, and when sent to the Vienna clinic was treated with drugs with unpleasant side effects and painful electric shocks. It is hard to know in retrospect, but one interpretation is that in this case Wagner-Jauregg had mistaken an organic brain injury for shell shock (Roth, 1988). In 1920 he was indicted for employing treatments which could be construed as torture. Among those who were called to testify on the first day of the hearing was Sigmund Freud.

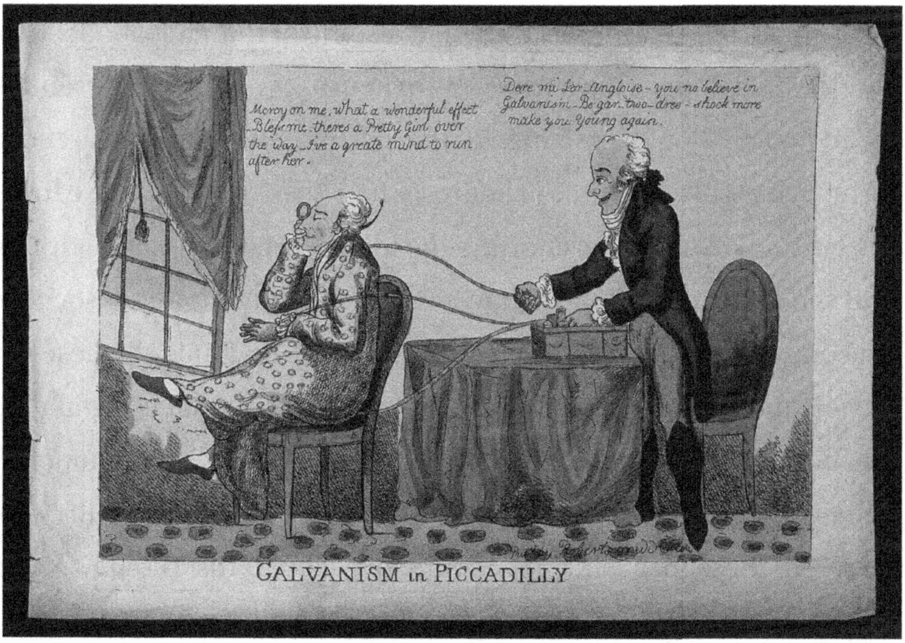

Figure 3-2: *Although the use of electrical treatments received a kind of notoriety during World War I, it had a history going back long before. In the 18th century it had a certain popularity, largely as a bogus treatment, as seen in this drawing depicting a wealthy patient looking out the window while a 'doctor' applied a galvanic current. Medical treatment with electricity was performed in London's Middlesex Hospital beginning in about 1767. It began to be considered a mainstream, if not yet very specific, mode of therapy in the mid-19th century with the work at Guy's Hospital by Dr. Golding Bird, who used it for conditions including paralyses, Sydenham's chorea (St. Virus' Dance), hysteria, and opiate overdoses. It was often used to diminish pain from various conditions but faced substantial skepticism by the beginning of the 20th century (Stillings, 1975). The use of electrical treatments for shell shock in World War I, then, was not a new technique; what was new was the widespread military mis-application of it in a purposely painful and punitive manner in order to motivate soldiers to return to the front.*

Freud's testimony:

As we described earlier, Freud's thinking about violence and society's (not always successful) function in controlling it had evolved during World War I. He had also been thinking about shell shock, which led him to a new view of neuroses, which he presented at an international meeting in the fall of 1918. One of Freud's formulations of the source of neuroses had been that they arose from the tension between the efforts of the id to express instinctual drives and the endeavors of the ego to shape this expression in a socially acceptable manner (Figure 3-3). He came to think of these as 'peacetime' neuroses. In contrast, the experience of military training and combat is so potent that it creates a new 'warlike' ego model of behavior, and shell shock could be seen as a conflict inside the ego between these peaceful and combative standards (Freud, 1919; Coblence, 2022). In his view, this is so stressful that a soldier may unconsciously develop a 'flight into illness', and manifest the many symptoms such as blindness, anxiety and depression. He was arguing, then, that a shell-shocked soldier was indeed suffering from a condition that originated in the mind, but required treatment, and should not be seen as a malingerer.

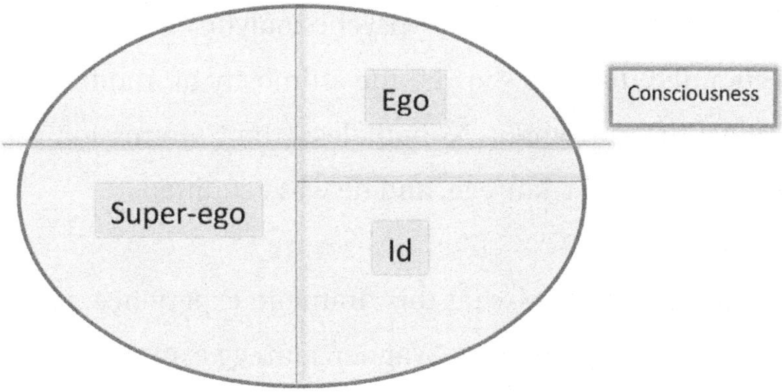

Figure 3-3: *Freud's 'structural' model, which came to fruition in the 1920s, pictures a 'psychic apparatus' with three interacting components: the id, which is the unconscious source of instinctual drives; the superego, which promotes moral standards acquired from parents and society, and enforces them by criticism and prohibitions; and the ego, which is reality-based and mediates the interaction of superego and id.*

Freud expressed this view on the first day of testimony. He went on to say that electric shock procedures, which he described as 'machine guns behind the front' were not designed to treat the soldier's neurosis, but rather to return him to battle as soon as possible (Scharf, 2022). Although he was critical of the electrical treatments, he did not speak negatively about Wagner-Jauregg as an individual, and emphasized that there was no issue of dereliction of duty (Eissler, 1979). Toward the end he also commented that it should be remembered that the doctors practicing these techniques were under 'military command', compromising their role as physicians. He suggested that they may have been guided by what he described as the German tendency to follow through with their intentions at all costs (Coblence, 2022).

The following day saw testimony by a number of psychiatrists who assailed Freud and the psychoanalytic method. Freud later responded that this showed the animosity of traditional psychiatry against his movement. Nonetheless, the Commission report spoke highly of Wagner-Jauregg, and he was acquitted.

It is hard to picture what this dramatic experience was like for the two men. In his memoirs, Wagner-Jauregg expressed feeling hurt by Freud's testimony, though Freud had avoided direct criticism of him. One can speculate that Freud felt the awkwardness of his position in giving testimony about his colleague, with whom he had gone to medical school and later training, even though he was hostile to psychoanalysis. It was also ironic that Freud had now been sitting in judgment on a man who had strongly recommended that he not be given a professorship in 1899 and gave him but a tepid review in 1919 (Chapter Two). Both men were now in their early sixties, and this was to be their last significant interaction. As Whitrow (1990) points out, the remarkable thing was that after the Commission they continued to express friendship for each other, in the form for instance of exchanging birthday cards in which they referred to each other with the German familiar word 'Du'.

Wagner-Jauregg and malaria treatment of dementia paralytica

As we mentioned in Chapter One, while working in Leidesdorf's clinic in his first years in a psychiatric setting, Wagner-Jauregg had noticed that some of his patients seemed to improve in their mental symptoms after they had experienced febrile illnesses including erysipelas and typhoid fever. Notably among these was a woman admitted with a severe psychosis, who caught typhoid; afterwards her mental status became normal, though later her original symptoms reappeared. The idea that febrile illnesses might at least temporarily improve mental illness was not new. It had its roots in antiquity with the Greek physicians Hippocrates and Galen. Moreover, there had been earlier reports (Koster, 1848; Nasse, 1864) of psychoses improving after patients had suffered from malaria. Intrigued by this notion, in 1877 he wrote an article 'On the effect of feverish disease on psychoses' in which he presented his cases and speculated about purposefully infecting patients as a treatment for mental illness. By 1888 he went so far as purposely infecting some of his patients with streptococci bacteria from people suffering from erysipelas. He induced plenty of febrile illnesses, but no obvious improvement in their psychoses. Years later, in his Nobel Prize lecture he called the experiments 'unfortunate', and added that he paused the work because 'I also hardly had the authority then to carry on with them' (Wagner-Jauregg, 1927).

In 1890 he came across what initially seemed like a safer approach. The German physician Robert Koch had developed tuberculin, material from the bacteria causing tuberculosis, which he believed might prevent and treat the illness (see Appendix). Wagner-Jauregg was able to obtain some samples of tuberculin, and reasoned that by giving it to his patients he would be able to induce fevers without actually causing infections. He administered it in 1890 and 1891, and in two cases there was improvement in psychotic symptoms. The work was soon discontinued, however. At the time he commented that the benefits of tuberculin were slow to appear, and that the hospital in Graz was designed for acute patients, who had to be discharged relatively quickly without long-term observation. In later years he wrote that he was also concerned that the toxicity of tuberculin had been underestimated, and that severe reactions and even death were being reported.

By the time Jauregg returned to Vienna in 1893, safer regimens with tuberculin had been established, and he resumed his studies. He had noticed that his successes tended to be in patients with dementia paralytica, suspected and later confirmed to be a delayed consequence of syphilis, causing psychosis, neurological symptoms, and wasting (see Appendix). At the time, it accounted for perhaps twenty percent of institutionalized patients, and was almost invariably fatal within three or four years.

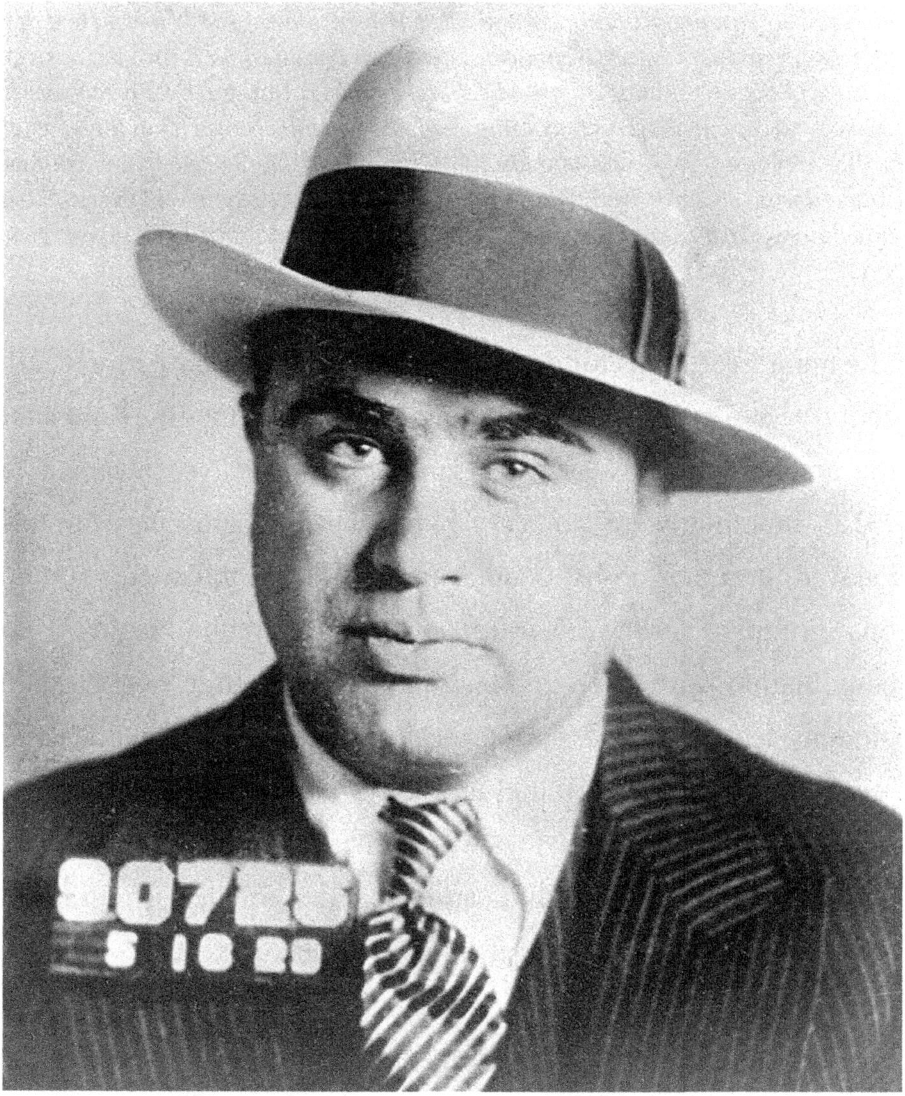

Figure 3-4: *A famous illustrative case of dementia paralytica, though it occurred a little later than this point in the narrative, was that of the Chicago gangster Al Capone. Shown here in a 1929 mugshot, he was able to evade the FBI, but not the IRS nor the consequences of syphilis in the nervous system. He was first diagnosed with syphilis, which he had likely had for some time, upon entering the federal prison system at age 33 in 1932. For a few years his behavior remained intact, and at Alcatraz he was known for his musical talents on the banjo while playing with other prisoners in a group called the Rock Islanders. Then gradually he showed unusual behavior (wearing winter outdoor clothes in heated rooms), had*

increasingly emotional outbursts, and was uncooperative. By 1938 it was clear that he was becoming progressively disoriented and confused, and the diagnosis of neurosyphilis was made. He was discharged from prison for health reasons in 1939. By 1942 penicillin was becoming available and he received it but the damage to his nervous system was already too severe. He experienced hallucinations, suffered from seizures. and deteriorated physically. By 1946 he was described as functioning like a 12 year old, and he died of complications of a stroke at age 48 in 1947.

The main treatments for dementia paralytica in the late nineteenth century were inorganic preparations of mercury or iodine (and later the arsenic-based drugs Salvarsan in 1910 and Neosalvarsan in 1912), but they were not very beneficial by themselves for this delayed form of syphilis. Wagner-Jauregg began to concentrate on this group. Those who received the tuberculin regimen in combination with mercury and iodine did better overall than patients who had not had fever therapy, although many later relapsed. Those whose initial febrile responses had been greatest seemed to have been the ones who clinically did better. In 1909 he presented these results to an audience at a medical congress in Budapest who remained largely unconvinced.

Wagner-Jauregg had noticed that the patients with more lasting benefits had later by chance experienced another febrile illness, and began to wonder whether there might be a treatable infectious disease which could be given to the paralytic patients. Malaria seemed particularly suitable for this purpose. It produced intermittent periods of fever, and moreover, in this pre-antibiotic era, it was essentially the only infectious disease for which an effective treatment—quinine—was available (see Appendix).

Wagner-Jauregg's opportunity came along during World War I. In June 1917 he came across a soldier who had contracted malaria in Macedonia. Malaria can produce a wide range of psychiatric symptoms, and indeed was among the leading causes of psychiatric symptoms of soldiers in the Balkans, which may explain his transfer to Wagner-Jauregg's clinic in Vienna. During a febrile episode Wagner-Jauregg obtained blood samples, and injected them into two patients with dementia paralytica; he then took blood from them and gave it to additional patients. In this manner, nine patients were treated, of whom six seemed to improve, although three later relapsed. All patients were later treated with quinine for their malaria.

The initial success of the treatments was tempered in 1918 by a reminder of the potentially lethal consequences of malaria. Wagner-Jauregg stumbled upon a particularly potent strain, causing what is known as malaria tropica, and three out of four patients died even after quinine treatment (Whitrow, 1993). These were not reported, and it is thought that Wagner-Jauregg had not microscopically checked the donor's blood to determine the type of *Plasmodium* which was present (Fiolet and Daey Ouwens, 2020). By 1920, he had obtained a somewhat safer strain, and the work resumed.

Wagner-Jauregg now designed studies in which patients alternately admitted to the hospital received either malaria therapy alone or malaria therapy followed by Neosalvarsan, and found the combination more effective, producing full remissions in 48.5%

compared to only 25% with febrile therapy alone. It also became clear that treating patients early, when they first came to the clinic, produced much better results than with inpatients. In one study of 38 outpatients, 84.8% had full remissions and 12.1% a partial remission; only one went on to require admission to the asylum (Wagner-Jauregg, 1927).

By 1921 he had treated over 150 patients. Insofar as dementia paralytica treated conventionally was almost invariably fatal, his work was well received, even though up to 20 percent of patients succumbed to malaria even with quinine treatment (Vogel, 2013; Daey Ouwens et al., 2017). Following larger case series in other German hospitals, malaria treatment for dementia paralytica became common throughout Europe, the Americas, Japan and South Africa. In 1926, a review of over 2000 cases in the international literature reported that about one quarter (27.5%) were greatly improved and another quarter (25.6%) were moderately benefitted (Brown, 2000). In 1927 Wagner-Jauregg was awarded the Nobel Prize for developing malaria therapy.

In later years, Wagner-Jauregg and others continued to speculate about chemical or physical alternatives for raising body temperature. Injections of sulfur or milk produced some success (Kragh, 2013). In the 1930s, an American group found that placing patients in a heated cabinet, the 'hypertherm' could raise body temperature up to 40 degrees Celsius, with beneficial results comparable to malaria therapy (Young, 2015). Both methods continued to be used until the 1940s and the advent of penicillin, which was much more effective, and soon became the preferred treatment (Mendelson, 2020).

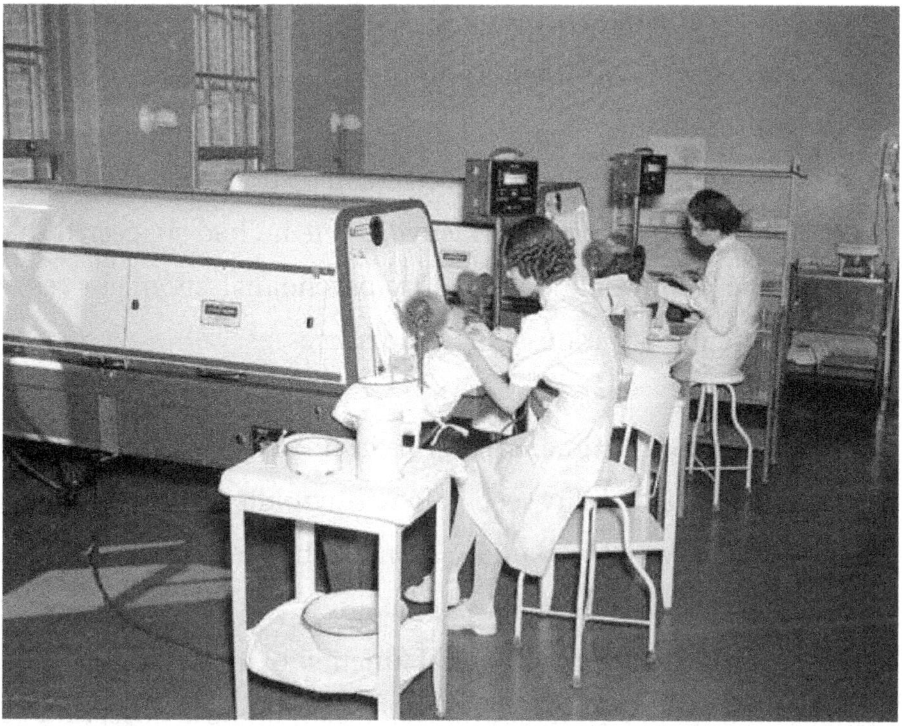

Figure 3-5: *Patients being treated with hypertherm cabinets, New Orleans, 1937.*

Wagner-Jauregg and endocrine treatments

Wagner-Jauregg, perhaps stimulated by his earlier success with cretinism and goiter (Chapter One), also explored various endocrine treatments in the 1920s. At the time, there was a growing interest in the relation of hormone function and psychiatric illness, derived from several sources. The American neurosurgeon Harvey Cushing had noted that overactivity of the parathyroid glands was often associated with psychoses. (To this day, medical students are taught that the symptoms of hyperparathyroidism include 'bones, stones and psychotic moans', referring to decreased bone density, kidney stones, as well as hallucinations or thought disorders.) Similarly he associated the changes in pituitary function during pregnancy with mental disorders in the perinatal period. In response to Freud's 1901 book *The Psychopathology of Everyday Life* he had suggested that many of the abnormalities noted by psychoanalysts might result from dysfunction of various endocrine processes.

Starting in 1908, Maxime Laignel-Lavastine, a French physician, emphasized the irritability seen in hyperthyroidism as well as mood changes and psychotic manifestations of hypothyroidism. As his work continued he described personality types or temperaments which he associated with abnormal function of the ovaries, adrenal glands and pituitary. As a natural conclusion of these observations, he believed that extracts of these various organs might be used therapeutically in psychiatric illness.

These thoughts were soon put into practice. In the early 1920s, Edward Strecker and Baldwin Keys in Philadelphia speculated that depression in midlife might result from decreased sexual endocrine function, and reported improvement after giving patients ovarian extracts. It was in this climate that Wagner-Jauregg became more aware of the possibilities of such treatments. He had come to believe that some young psychotic patients seemed to have delayed puberty, and reported that administration of both thyroid and ovarian preparations resulted in a decrease in their symptoms. Similarly, psychiatrists at St. Anne's Hospital in Paris reported benefits of androgen injections in psychoses.

In the 19th century, sexual excitement and excessive masturbation had often been thought to lead to a variety of disorders, including epilepsy. Indeed, in 1857, Charles Locock, a London physician who was interested in epilepsy occurring around the time of the menses, had used potassium bromide, which decreased sexual drive, as a treatment. It was later tried in other forms of seizure disorders; as a result, a misguided Victorian belief about sex led to the development of a class of anticonvulsants which remained in widespread use until the development of the barbiturate drugs in the early 20th century. Excessive masturbation was also thought to result in psychoses in males. As a consequence, Wagner-Jauregg sterilized some patients by surgically interrupting the vas deferens in the testes, again believing that he had achieved some therapeutic success.

Wagner-Jauregg, then, was participating in a widespread interest in endocrine processes in psychiatry in the 1920s, which moved into a number of other areas including studies of glucose metabolism and insulin function. Interest in the field diminished over time, later being stimulated again with the discovery of cortisol in 1947 and studies of its apparently disturbed regulation in depression in the 1960s and 1970s (Shorter and Fink, 2009). Wagner-Jauregg's work also carried other themes, however. In addition to touching on lingering Victorian notions of sexuality, with implied disapproval of the allegedly sexual sources of some psychoses, his treatments may have been precursors to his later very public advocacy of sterilization of 'degenerates' in the late 1930s.

REFERENCES for CHAPTER THREE

BBC: Inside out: Shell shock, 2004.
https://www.bbc.co.uk/insideout/extra/series- 1/shell_shocked.sh tml (Accessed February 7, 2022).

Bogousslavsky, J.:_Hysteria after Charcot: back to the future. Front. Neurol. Neurosci. 29: 137-161, 2011.
https://pubmed.ncbi.nlm.nih.gov/20938153/

Brown, E.M.: Why Wagner-Jauregg won the Nobel Prize for discovering malaria therapy for general paresis of the insane. Hist. Psychiatry 9: 371-382, 2000.

Coblence, F.: Freud and War, in Arts & Societes letter of seminar.
https://www.sciencespo.fr/artsetsocietes/en/archives/1187
(Accessed February 9, 2022).

Crocq, M-A.: From shell shock and war neurosis to posttraumatic stress disorder: a history of psychotraumatology. Dialogues Clin. Neurosci. 2: 47-55, 2000.

Danto, E.A.: Trauma and the state with Sigmund Freud as Witness. Int. J. Law Psychiatry 48: 50-56, 2016. https://pubmed.ncbi.nlm.nih.gov/27324417/

Eissler, K.R.: *Freud und Wagner-Jauregg vor der Kommission zur Erhebung militarischer Pflichtverletzungen*. Locker Verlag, Vienna, 1979.

Fiolet, A.T.L. and Daey Ouwens, I.M.: History of neurology: treatment evaluation takes time. World Neurology, Oct/Nov 2020. https://worldneurologyonline.com/article/treatment-evaluation-takes-time/ (Accessed February 20, 2022).

Freud, S.: *Thoughts for the Times on War and Death,* 1916. https://www.loc.gov/exhibits/freud/ex/175.html

Freud, S.: Introduction to *Psycho-Analysis and War Neuroses* (1919), *Standard Edition,* vol. 17, p. 209.

Freud, S.: *Civilization and its Discontents.* W.W. Norton & Co., 2021 (Original text in 1930).

Freud Library 12: Freud, S.: *Civilization Society and Religion.* Penguin, 1985. https://www.amazon.com/Library-Civilization-Society-Religion-Pelican/dp/0140217452

Friedman, M.J.:_PTSD history and overview. U.S. Dept. of Veterans Affairs, National Center for PTSD.
https://www.ptsd.va.gov/professional/treat/essentials/history_ptsd.asp (Accessed January 8, 2021).

Gay, P. (ed), Freud, S. (author): *The Freud Reader.* W.W. Norton, 1995.
https://www.amazon.com/Freud-Reader-Sigmund/dp/0393314030/ref=sr_1_1?crid=WK07T6ZQO6UE&dchild=1&keywords=project+for+a+scientific+psychology+freud&qid=1611247644&sprefix=project+for+a+scientifi%2Caps%2C208&sr=8-1

Freud, S.: *Thoughts for the Times on War and Death.*
https://www.loc.gov/exhibits/freud/ex/175.html

Freud, S.: *Mourning and Melancholia.* Collected Papers, Vol. IV, 152-170, 1917.

Kaufmann F. Die planmäβige Heilung komplizierter psychogener Bewegungsstörungen bei Soldaten in einer Sitzung. *In: Feldärtz Beilage Münch Med Wochenschr.* 1916;63:802ff.

Kleinert, R., in: Julius Wagner-Jauregg, in Whonamedit? A dictionary of medical eponyms.
https://www.whonamedit.com/doctor.cfm/2753.html Accessed January 18, 2022.

Koster, F: Quomodo in insaniam valeatfebr. Intermittens, Bonn, 1848 (Thesis at the University of Bonn).

Kragh JV. 'Fumbling in the Dark'. Malaria, sulfosin and metallosal in the treatment of mental disorders in Denmark, 1917-1937". In: Volker Roelcke & Hans-Walter Schmuhl, editors:*Heroische Therapien.* Göttingen. Wallensteins Verlag. 2013: 102-115.

Mendelson, W.B.: *The Curious History of Medicines in Psychiatry.* Pythagoras Press, 2020.
https://www.amazon.com/dp/B083ZRMCW1

Mendelson, W.B.: *Trial by Fire: World War II and the Founders of Modern Neuroscience and Psychopharmacology.* Pythagoras Press, 2021.
https://www.amazon.com/dp/B08X1MRVXJ

Nasse, W.: 'NeueBeobachtungenfiberdenEinflussdesWechselfieber saufdasIresein',Alg.Z. Psychiat.,1864,21:1-46

O'Neill, A. in Statistica: Number of casualties and fatalities during the Battle of the Somme in 1916.
https://www.statista.com/statistics/1022625/casualty-fatalities-statistics-battle-somme-1916/ (Accessed February 7, 2022).

Roth, N.: Freud as an expert witness. The discussion of war neuroses between Freud and Wagner-Jauregg, by K.R. Eissler (Book Review). J. Am. Acad. Psychoanalysis, N.Y., 16: 259, 1988. https://www.proquest.com/openview/ad8b90080e9ca33fba77bc6f7da135c1/1?pq-origsite=gscholar&cbl=1820984

Scharf, M.: Neurotics or shirkers? In The World of the Hapsburgs: The First World War. https://ww1.habsburger.net/en/chapters/neurotics-or-shirkers (Accessed January 8, 2022)

Shaw, B.: Historical context for the writings of Sigmund Freud. Columbia College: The Core Curriculum. https://www.college.columbia.edu/core/content/writings-sigmund-freud/context (Accessed January 9, 2021)

Shorter, E. and Fink, M.: *Endocrine Psychiatry: Solving the Riddle of Melancholia.* Oxford University Press, 2010.

Stillings, D.: A survey of the history of electrical stimulation for pain to 1900. Med. Instrumentation 9: 255-259, 1975. https://europepmc.org/article/med/1102872

Vogel, G.: Malaria as a lifesaving therapy. Science 342: 686, 2013. https://www.science.org/doi/10.1126/science.342.6159.686

Wagner-Jauregg J (1887). Über die Einwirkung fieberhafter Erkrankungen auf Psychosen[On the effect of feverish disease on psychoses]. Jahrbuch Psychiat. Neurol. 7:94-131.

Wagner-Jauregg, J.: Nobel lecture: The treatment of dementia paralytica by malaria inoculation. https://www.nobelprize.org/prizes/medicine/1927/wagner-jauregg/lecture/ (Accessed February 17, 2022).

Whitrow, M.: Freud and Wagner-Jauregg: A historiographical study. Psychiatric Bulletin 14: 356-358, 1990.

Young M.: *Encyclopedia of Asylum Therapeutics, 1750-1950.* Jefferson, North Carolina: McFarland & Company. 2015: 131.

CHAPTER FOUR: THE TROUBLED YEARS LEADING TO WORLD WAR II

Freud and the Gestapo

As we described in Chapter Three, by 1930 Freud was trying to formulate the role of violent impulses in society, as exemplified by *Civilization and its Discontents.* Once again he began to experience the pathway to war, with the growing political influence and violence of the Nazis. In 1932, Albert Einstein wrote him from Berlin, asking if he thought war was so inherent in human nature that it is inevitable, or whether it can be prevented. In a famous reply, Freud emphasized both the depth to which we have instincts for violence, but also the hope for human culture which can 'master our instinctive life'. In Freud's words, 'He (Einstein) understands as much about psychology as I (Freud) do about physics, so we had a very pleasant talk' (Ninivaggi, 2012).

Einstein and Freud followed very different paths after this exchange. Shortly after Hitler became Chancellor of Germany in 1933, Einstein fled to England and later the U.S., in an exodus that included many other luminaries including the psychologists Erik Erikson and Erich Fromm. Freud chose to stay in Vienna. He had been diagnosed with cancer of the jaw a decade earlier, and was determined to die in Vienna, where he would 'disappear from this world with decency'. By that time Freud was experiencing the growing persecution firsthand. The book burnings which took place beginning in May 1933 were devoted to 'un-German' works, of which Freud's were so high on the list that a special 'fire-oath' denouncing 'overvaluation of sexual activity' was recited as his books were thrown into the flames. Freud is said to have commented at the time: 'What progress we are making. In the Middle Ages they would have burned me; nowadays they are content with burning my books (Reef, 2001).

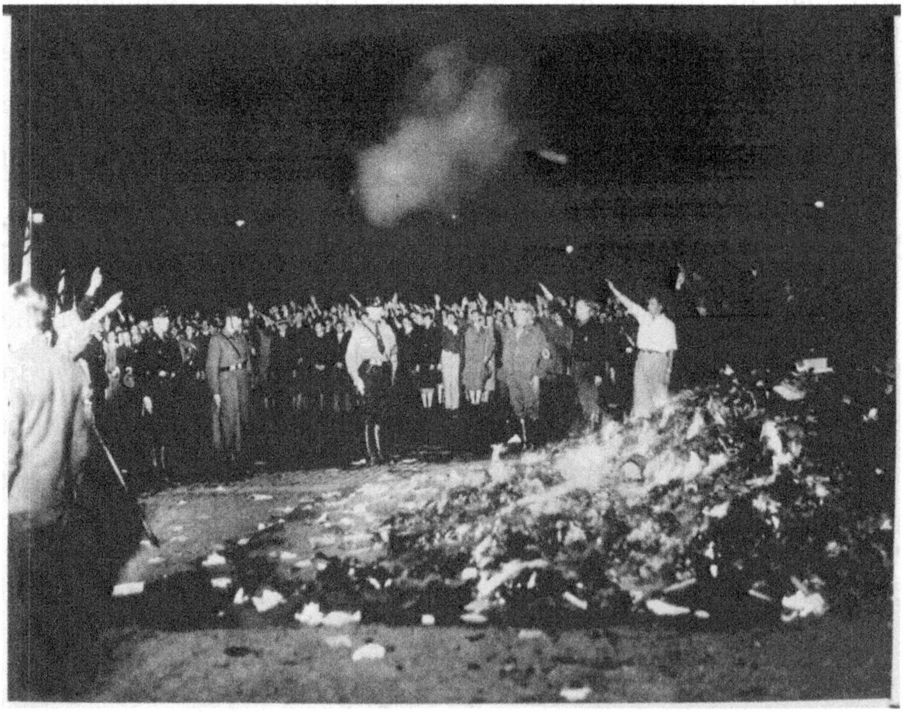

Figure 4-1: *Participants give the Nazi salute during a book burning in 1933. The most well-known episode was on May 10, 1933, in which burnings occurred in 34 cities, destroying perhaps 25,000 books. In Berlin and some other cities, the*

proceedings were broadcast 'live' on the radio. Besides Freud, authors who were targeted included Karl Marx, socialists such as Berthold Brecht and August Bebel, and the German novelists Thomas Mann and Erich Maria Remarque. American writers included Jack London, Theodore Dreiser, and Ernest Hemingway, as well as Helen Keller, presumably because of her support for the disabled.

The day after the German annexation of Austria in March 1938, the 82-year-old Freud's home was raided by the Gestapo, who took his money, valuables and passport. Left with little but his sense of humor, he commented at the time 'I never received as much for a house call' (U.S. Holocaust Museum, 2021). Freud's sons had already left, but

the Gestapo arrested his daughter Anna, who took with her a bottle containing a lethal dose of Veronal (a barbiturate) in case she were to be tortured (Tucker, 2019). She was later released after protests by two ex-patients, William Bullitt, the American ambassador to France, and Princess Marie Bonaparte, great-granddaughter of Napoleon, as well as a phone call from the American consul in Vienna to the Gestapo during her interrogation.

Freud was now committed to exile, but the problem was obtaining permission. Fortunately, help came from several sources. One was once again his princess-patient, who paid the Nazis a considerable amount of money to allow him to leave (Latson, 2015). He is also said to have obtained help from an unlikely source, Anton Sauerwald, a German official who had been appointed to oversee Freud's possessions and publishing business. Sauerwald was a 40-year-old chemist, and he himself read some of Freud's works and came to respect him. He sold some of Freud's possessions to raise money, which he used to pay for favorable action on visas for him and some of his family (Cohen, 2012). The story is a complicated one—he was a Nazi whose hobby was bomb-making, and after the war he was charged with war crimes including stealing the family's assets. A letter from Anna Freud in his support ultimately aided in his release from jail.

On June 4, 1938, Freud was allowed to take the Orient Express to Paris, as a first stop on the way to London. Before he could board, the Gestapo required him to sign a document freeing them from any blame for his treatment. They perhaps did not appreciate his sense of humor when he wrote 'I can heartily recommend the Gestapo to anyone' (Cohen, 2012).

Once in London, Freud continued to be troubled by cancer; Sauerwald, who had come to visit him, arranged for his Vienna doctor to travel there to perform an operation which Freud thought extended his life by a year. In his remaining time he was very productive. He saw patients in a room in his new Hampstead home which was designed to resemble his old office in Vienna, complete with the original couch. During this period he received visits from luminaries such as H.G. Wells, Salvador Dali, and Virginia Woolf. He completed his long-unfinished book *Moses and Monotheism*, and a synopsis of his lifetime's work, *An Outline of Psychoanalysis*, which came out posthumously. When asked how he had managed to do so much in the past year, his reply was 'Thank the Fuhrer' (Cohen,

2012). He died three weeks after war was declared in September 1939.

Wagner-Jauregg and racial hygiene

As described in Chapter One, when Wagner-Jauregg stepped down from being director of the clinic at the General Hospital, he remained very active. In addition to improvements in the technique of febrile therapy, he also expanded its application beyond dementia paralytica, to include work on schizophrenia and mood disorders (Whitrow, 1993). In doing so, one could see a progression from the man who in 1890 had ceased studies of tuberculin for some years after reports of severe reactions, to one who persisted after his own initial patients died of malaria tropica in 1918, and then to one who after 1928 advocated a treatment with a mortality of up to 20 percent (Vogel, 2013; Daey Ouwens et al., 2017) for psychiatric illnesses which, though they cause substantial suffering, produce lower death rates. There was also a progression from the young man who had married a Jewish woman to an older one who became more and more vocal about his views on what came to be known as racial hygiene (the belief that 'inferior' races might contaminate German 'racial purity').

These were not new ideas for Wagner-Jauregg, or for his culture. The belief that hereditary defects could over time lead to corruption of communities or even whole countries was expressed in many ways during the late 19th century (Pick, 1989). The allegedly harmful role of 'degenerates' in society was widely accepted in Austrian psychiatry, and as early as 1893, upon his return to Vienna from Graz, Wagner-Jauregg had declared that 'the majority [of degenerates] ended up in lunatic asylums or prisons, or else became anarchists and were responsible for such horrors as the Paris commune' (Marx, 1994). As we described in Chapter Three, during World War I, it was widely thought in the Vienna clinics that shell shock was primarily a disorder of degenerates, and in the 1920s Wagner-Jauregg had practiced sterilization on psychotic youths, believing that their condition resulted from excessive masturbation. It was but a small step, then, for him to support involuntary sterilization of the mentally ill and lawbreakers, and he began to do so in public forums.

By 1935 Wagner-Jauregg was active in the Austrian Anthropological Society (Holmes and Silverman, 2009), and he became president of the Austrian League for Racial Regeneration and Heredity, supporting forced sterilization of persons considered to be inferior (Loscher, 2007; Jacobsen et al., 2009). He was openly antisemitic (Shorter and Healy, 2007; Gartlehner and Stepper, 2012) and he supported the Nazis even before the German annexation of Austria in 1938. Soon afterwards he applied to join the party. He was initially turned down on the grounds that his first wife had been Jewish, and some have speculated on whether one of the roots of his antisemitism may have grown from that extremely unhappy marriage (Whitrow, 1993). He re-applied a few months before his death, and was honored in the obituaries of the Nazi press. After he passed away, the text of a book written for a broader public, *On the Human Lifespan,* was discovered on his desk and published the next year. In it he gave his full support to the German racial protection laws.

REFERENCES for CHAPTER FOUR

Cohen, D.: *Escape of Sigmund Freud.* Abrams Press, 2012. https://www.amazon.com/Escape-Sigmund-Freud-David-Cohen/dp/1590206738

Daey, O. et al.: Malaria fever therapy for general paresis of the insane: a historical cohort study. European Neurology 78: 56-62, 2017. https://worldneurologyonline.com/article/treatment-evaluation-takes-time/

Freud, S.: *Civilization and its Discontents.* W.W. Norton & Co., 2021 (Original text in 1930).357-359, 2012.

Gartlehner, G. and Stepper, K.: Julius Wagner-Jauregg: pyrothrapy, simultanmethode, and 'racial hygiene'. J. Royal Soc. Med. 105: 357-259, 2012. https://www.ncbi.nlm.nih.gov/pmc/articles/PMC3423136/

Latson, J.: Why Freud chose Nazi Germany over America. Time, May 6, 2015. https://time.com/3840374/freud-birthday-anniversary-history/

Loscher, M.: Eugenics and Catholicism in Interwar Austria. "*Blood And Homeland": Eugenics And Racial Nationalism in Central And Southeast Europe, 1900-1940.* Budapest: Central European University Press, 2007.

Marx, O.M.: Review of 'Magda Whitrow. *Julius Wagner-Jauregg (1857-1940).* Isis 85: 719, 1994. https://www.journals.uchicago.edu/doi/10.1086/357038 (Accessed February 9, 2022).

Ninivaggi, F.J.: Why War? Psychology Today, May 26, 2012. https://www.psychologytoday.com/us/blog/envy/201205/why-war

Pick, D.: *Faces of Degeneration: a European Disorder, c. 1948-1919.* Cambridge University Press, Cambridge and New York, 1989.

Reef, C.: *Sigmund Freud: Pioneer of the Mind.* Clarion, New York, NY, 2001.

Shorter, E. and Healy, D.: *Shock Therapy: a history of electroconvulsive treatment in mental illness.* Rutgers University Press, 2007, p. 20.

Tucker, N.: Freud's last days in Vienna as Nazis approached. Library of Congress Blog, September 23, 2019. https://blogs.loc.gov/loc/2019/09/freuds-last-days-in-vienna-as-nazis-approached/

United States Holocaust Memorial Museum, Washington, D.C.: Sigmund Freud. Accessed January 25, 2021. https://encyclopedia.ushmm.org/content/en/article/sigmund-freud

Wagner-Jauregg, J.: *Ueber die menschliche Lebersdauer* (On the human lifespan). Duetscher Alpenverlag, Innsbruck, 1941.

Whitrow, M.: Julius Wagner-Jauregg (1857-1940). J. Med. Biography 1: 137-143, 1993. https://journals.sagepub.com/doi/abs/10.1177/096777209300100302?journalCode=jmba

CHAPTER FIVE: SUMMARY AND CONCLUSIONS

In some ways, Freud and Wagner-Jauregg had very similar backgrounds: both were born and died within about a year of each other, were immersed in Austrian culture of the era, with similar medical training in Vienna and exposure to the same remarkable teachers such as Ernst von Brücke and Salomon Stricker. Both initially had similar aspirations to go into internal medicine, but ultimately became psychiatrists.

On the other hand, it could be argued that in some senses the experiences of Freud and Wagner-Jauregg were very different. Wagner-Jauregg came from a patrician family, which later became titled, and attended a secondary school known for teaching the children of the highborn. There is no reason to think that his various career moves were influenced by money, and indeed from the beginning, even in his first appointment in psychiatry under Leidesdorf, he had room and board and a reasonable salary. In contrast, Freud was the son of an unsuccessful merchant, had attended a public school, and was painfully aware of his finances. This consideration had led his mentor Ernst von Brücke to urge him in 1882 to leave his research studies of pathology in favor of clinical work at the General Hospital, though it too paid more poorly than Jauregg's position.

The two also seemed to take different approaches to becoming doctors. We know little about Wagner-Jauregg's decision, but he is said to have been fascinated with dissection in his secondary school years, and once entering the University of Vienna, took a relatively straightforward path to graduation. Freud, on the other hand, came out of secondary school speaking a number of languages, and had thought of going into law. He entered the university at the early age of 17, is said to have been influenced into more scientific interests by the writings of Goethe (who was himself both poet and scientist), and took a round-about course, studying philosophy and zoology before graduating a year later than usual.

Once Freud and Wagner-Jauregg had graduated, their hopes for careers in internal medicine frustrated, they went into psychiatry by very different routes. Jauregg, who had expressed no earlier interest in the field, by chance got a tip about a vacant position at the First Psychiatric Clinic from a professor acquaintance at a coffee house; with limited options available, he applied for it with alacrity. Freud's interest had a clearer evolution. In keeping with his earlier circuitous route to studying medicine, once at the General Hospital he worked in a variety of disciplines before being drawn to clinical neurology and psychiatry. Ultimately he was drawn to Charcot's work with hysteria, and after returning from his studies in Paris he continued to be stimulated by Joseph Breuer's work with Bertha Pappenheim.

Perhaps partly because of their different backgrounds but also their innate traits, as mature men they came across very differently in public settings. Wagner-Jauregg had 'an extraordinarily powerful personality', tended to dominate gatherings, often seemed gruff, and was later described in an obituary as a giant in body and spirit (Whitrow, 1993). Freud, was slim, professorial, and one has the impression that he generally had a quieter way of controlling meetings. He was also sensitive to criticism and quick to forcefully argue his points. He certainly had a quality which drew students to him, but also had little tolerance for their deviations from his ideas. In a therapeutic setting, some combination of his manner and the process of analysis produced tremendous loyalty from many of his patients, who as we have seen on several occasions made extraordinary efforts to help him when he was in difficult situations.

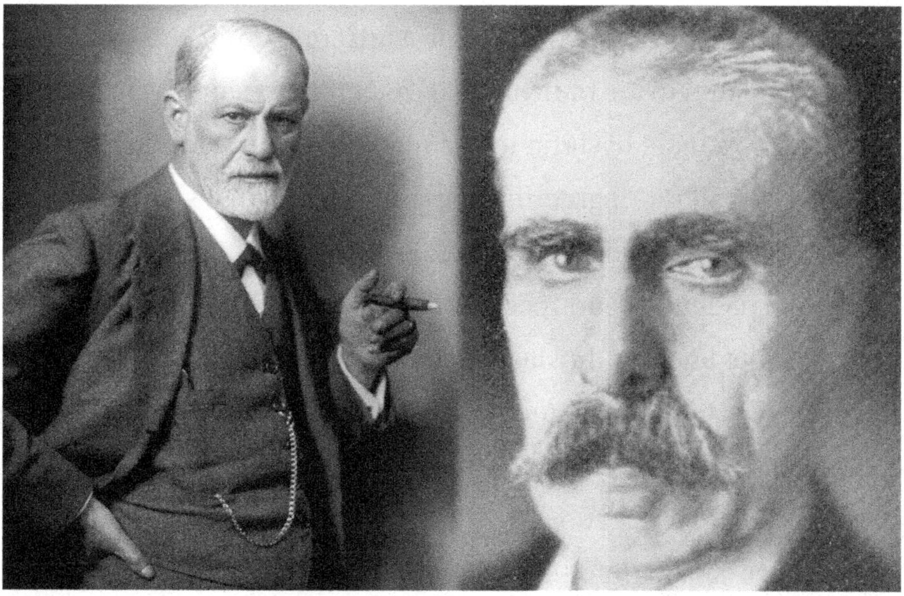

Figure 5-1: Left: *Freud in a photo taken by his son-in-law Max Halberstadt, 1921.* Right: *Wagner-Jauregg, undated but in the 1920's.*

Freud and Wagner-Jauregg also had very different trajectories in their attitudes and relations with universities. Though they both received the *Dozentur*, which allowed them to be unpaid lecturers in neuropathology at the same time in 1885, they then went on very different paths. Jauregg's was very much in the traditions of the formal institutions, and he rose rapidly, achieving an intermediate professorship in 1889 and full professorship in 1893. Freud, in contrast, felt differently about his relations to institutions. When awarded a fellowship to study with Charcot in 1885, he resigned from the General Hospital, though he could have taken a leave of absence. On his return in 1886, he established a private practice which he maintained for half a century. Having a university title was important to him in the sense that it allowed him to lecture, but the path was hard and slow, perhaps due to the antisemitism of the times and certainly related to his radical ideas. As but one example, in 1886 he gave a talk on male hysteria to the medical society, which offended Meynert to such a degree that he cancelled Freud's access to his clinic at the General Hospital. Apparently with the help of an illustrious patient, Freud received an intermediate professorship in 1889, despite an unenthusiastic letter from Wagner-Jauregg; he did not receive a full appointment until 26 years after Wagner-Jauregg did, in 1919. The historian Magda Whitrow points out that 'he was never a regular academic teacher' and believes that most biographies fail to mention that even these professorships were titular (Whitrow, 1990).

Perhaps one of the biggest differences between Freud and Wagner-Jauregg, however, may have been in their attitude toward a doctor's obligation to the patient and to society. It is perhaps not surprising that Wagner-Jauregg, who had benefitted from a patrician background, seemed to see himself much more as representing the society which had treated him so well. Thus, while Freud focused on shell shock as a neurosis which needed to be treated, Wagner-Jauregg emphasized methods to rapidly return his soldier-patients back to duty. There were, or course, broader issues at work than just their personalities. In a sense, Wagner-Jauregg was reflecting attitudes and worries throughout psychiatry in Austria-Hungary. During World War I, the Hapsburg monarchy was facing the collapse of a multinational empire and the emergence of national and regional antagonisms. It seems likely that the worry about these centrifugal forces helped shape the attitudes toward shell shock and its treatment (Hofer, 2011). Likewise, in Wagner-Jauregg's growing post-World War I interest in sterilizing 'degenerate' patients, and his later blatant advocacy of racial hygiene, he was coming to see himself more and more as an agent of the state. Nowhere was this made clearer than in *On the Human Lifespan*, where he wrote 'the production of a most favorable genotype was the task of the physician and the legislator as a racial hygienist' (Marx, 1994).

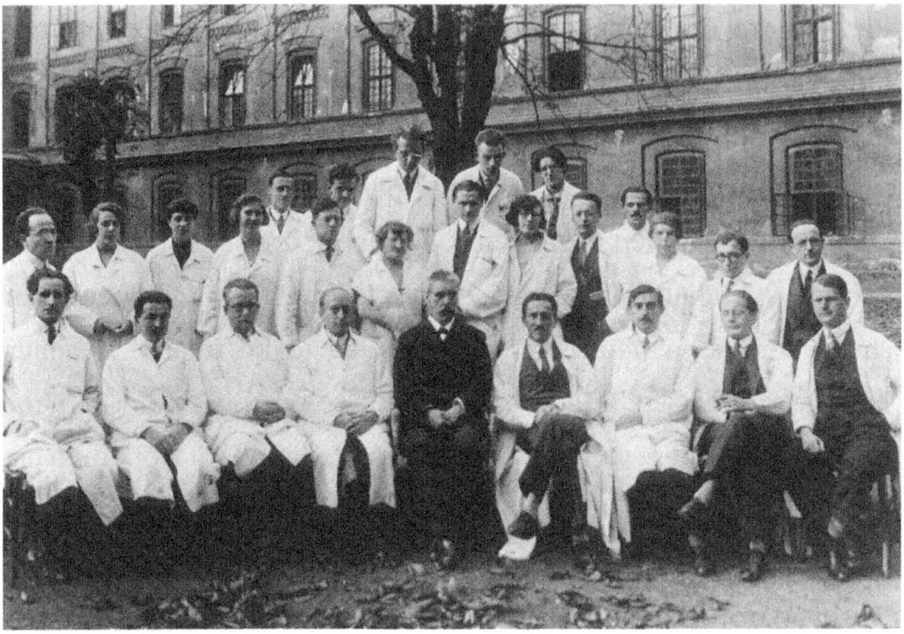

Figure 5-2: *Wagner-Jauregg and his staff, 1927. He is seen in center of the first row, wearing black.*

In contrast to Wagner-Jauregg, Freud's natural focus was on the obligation to the patient, perhaps in part reflecting his increasing alienation from the society in which he lived. As we described in Chapter Three, in the years after World War I he had concluded that the role of civilization in the formation of personality could be double-edged, either helping to control, or in some circumstances unleashing, the impulse toward violence. Moreover, politicians were authority figures, invoking all the reactions to father representations which he had considered at such length.

In a more immediate sense, Freud's distancing himself from the culture surrounding him was not surprising in view of the growing antisemitism in the 1920s. His biographer Peter Gay (1998) quotes him as saying in 1926:

> *"My language is German. My culture, my attainments are German. I considered myself German intellectually, until I noticed the growth of antisemitic prejudice in Germany and German Austria. Since that time, I prefer to call myself a Jew."*

This was a remarkable evolution in self-image in a man who had always proclaimed himself an atheist, although his cultural writings often turned to religion (Cooper-White, 2017), culminating in *Moses and Monotheism*, completed in the last year of his life.

What, then, was the bond between Freud and Wagner-Jauregg, aside from their common background in medical school and training in neuropathology? Perhaps they recognized that they were likely to continue to be in positions to influence each other's careers. Wagner-Jauregg, for instance, wrote letters regarding Freud's applications for a professorship in 1899 and 1919, while Freud was among the first to testify at the hearing on Wagner-Jauregg's treatment of shell shock in 1920. Freud was certainly not someone who was afraid of a fight with those who differed with him, as evidenced by his longstanding hostilities with Carl Jung, yet even though he disagreed with Wagner-Jauregg's treatments during the war, he did his best to be protective at the hearings. Perhaps he realized that they both were part of a small and very interactive psychiatric community in Vienna, and would be for some time to come. And perhaps they both recognized the brilliance in each other, though they disapproved of the directions in which it had taken them.

In their last two decades, they had little contact beyond formalities, and their differences continued to increase. Although Freud's fame flourished inside his profession, he became more and more isolated from his previous German/Austrian identity, and he ultimately died in exile. Wagner-Jauregg saw himself more and more affiliated with the rise of German fascism, and used his knowledge of medicine to further its promotion of racial hygiene. The practical applications of such thinking evolved into the horrors of the Third Reich. When the Third Reich later collapsed, his reputation died along with it.

REFERENCES for CHAPTER FIVE

Cooper-White, P.: Freud's Vienna circle, psychoanalysis and antisemitism. SCJR 12: 1-15, 2017.
https://www.facinghistory.org/holocaust-and-human-behavior/chapter-4/antisemitism-and-jewish-identity

Gay, P.: *Freud: A Life for Our Time* (New York: Norton, 1998), 448.

Hofer, H.-G.: Beyond Freud and Wagner-Jauregg: War, psychiatry and the Hapsburg army. Neuere Medizin- und Wissenschaftsgeschichte 26:49-71, 2011.
https://www.researchgate.net/publication/51656479_Beyond_Freud_and_Wagner-Jauregg_War_Psychiatry_and_the_Habsburg_Army

Jones, E.: *Sigmund Freud Life and Work, 1961, p. 233.*

Marx, O.M.: Review of 'Magda Whitrow: *Julius Wagner-Jauregg (1857-1940).* ISIS 85, 719, 1994.
https://www.journals.uchicago.edu/doi/10.1086/357038

Wagner-Jauregg, J.: *Ueber die menschliche Lebersdauer* (On the human lifespan). Duetscher Alpenverlag, Innsbruck, 1941.

Whitrow, M.: Freud and Wagner-Jauregg: A historiographical study. Psychiatric Bulletin 14: 356-358, 1990.

Whitrow, M.: *Julius Wagner-Jauregg (1857-1940).* Smith-Gordon, 1993.

APPENDIX

Although the focus of this book is on the interactions of Freud and Wagner-Jauregg, it may be helpful to look at the context in which they occurred. Certainly the role of three illnesses in the late 19th and early 20th century—malaria, syphilis and tuberculosis—clarifies the significance of Wagner-Jauregg's work. Similarly, the history of a different kind of affliction—antisemitism in France, Germany and Austria—gives context to a number of aspects of Freud's life.

Malaria, the 'Roman fever' across the centuries

Malaria, which is caused by microscopic *Plasmodium* protozoa transmitted by infected *Anopheles* mosquitos, has affected humans as far back as the New Stone Age, and currently infects about two hundred million people annually. Over the millennia, humans have developed genetic mutations to provide partial resistance, some of which result in present-day illnesses such as sickle cell disease and thalassemia. Malaria has affected human history in remarkable ways, hampering the construction of the Egyptian pyramids, contributing to the fall of Rome (where it was called 'Roman fever'), felling Renaissance princes, and hindering the British army in the South during the American Revolutionary War.

After a person is bitten by an infective mosquito, the *Plasmodium* protozoa begin a life cycle in which it goes through a series of stages and at different times is found in the liver and in the bloodstream, where it occupies red blood cells. Typically, signs of illness begin to appear in about 7-30 days, and at first may not be easily recognizable as malaria. Symptoms include intermittent fever and chills, sweating, jaundice, fatigue, muscular pains and headache. Psychiatric symptoms may appear as well. Irritability and insomnia are common, and in some cases confusion, memory disturbances and manic-like symptoms may appear. During the Balkan campaign in World War I, soldiers might be sidelined by confusional psychoses, which were only later understood to be associated with malaria when fever and other symptoms became more evident. Some patients may have diminished levels of consciousness progressing to coma accompanied by neurological deficits in what is known as 'cerebral malaria'.

Children are particularly susceptible to the more severe forms of malaria, and constitute about two-thirds of the deaths. Without treatment, people with malaria who survive may experience a second, often milder, episode a few months later, and despite partial immunity may have further episodes months or years later. Malaria can be caused by five species of the *Plasmodium* parasite, which differ in their severity of disease. *Plasmodium falciparum* produces the highest mortality, while *vivax*, which was used most extensively in malaria therapy for dementia paralytica after first trying more lethal strains, is the most common source of malaria infection around the world. Both, along with *P. ovale*, produce what is known as tertian malaria, in which fever episodes are most evident every second day, though this pattern is usually less clear in the clinic than in classical teaching (CDC, 2019).

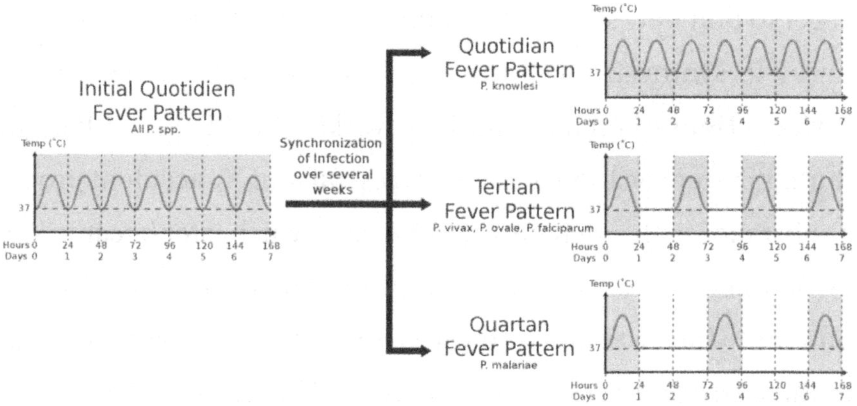

Figure A-1: *Fever patterns in malaria.*

The first signs of an effective treatment for malaria appeared in colonial South America. Legend had it that a feverish Amerindian drank water made bitter by the surrounding 'quina-quina' trees (now known as *Cinchona officinalis*), and found relief, and this became a common practice. In the seventeenth century, missionaries in the Peruvian Andes noted this, and began using it for malaria in the lowlands. Jesuit's Bark, as it was known, was taken to Europe, and quinine was identified as the active ingredient in 1820. Europeans, eager to import large quantities, were faced with efforts by South American countries to maintain their monopoly by preventing export of seeds or plants. Smuggled seeds eventually found their way to Europe. The Dutch, in particular, realized their value and sent them to Indonesia, where vast plantations led to their dominating the market, as they did for rubber as well.

By the mid-nineteenth century, the British, recognizing that malaria was making it much harder to maintain a worldwide empire, were eager to find new sources of quinine. One result was an effort to find a way to synthesize it at the Royal College of Chemistry. In 1857, William Henry Perkin, a student working in his home laboratory during Easter vacation, was unsuccessful, but by accident produced a substance with a rich purple color, and which later became known as aniline purple or mauveine. Although he had failed to make quinine, which was not synthesized until 1944, his discovery resulted in the formation of the synthetic dye industry, which later used the tools of synthetic organic chemistry to create medicines ranging from antibacterials to psychiatric drugs (Mendelson, 2020). Interestingly, some of these dye derivatives later became treatments for malaria; a yellow acridine dye evolved into quinacrine in 1931, followed by chloroquine in 1934 and hydroxychloroquine in 1955. (In contrast to these successful agents, a methylene blue derivative that was found to be ineffective for malaria went on in 1952 to play a major role in psychiatry as the first antipsychotic, chlorpromazine (Mendelson, 2020b)). Coming back to our narrative, however, when Wagner-Jauregg was considering purposely infecting patients with malaria in 1917, the synthetic antimicrobials were not yet developed, and malaria stood out among infectious diseases as the only one with a generally effective treatment, quinine.

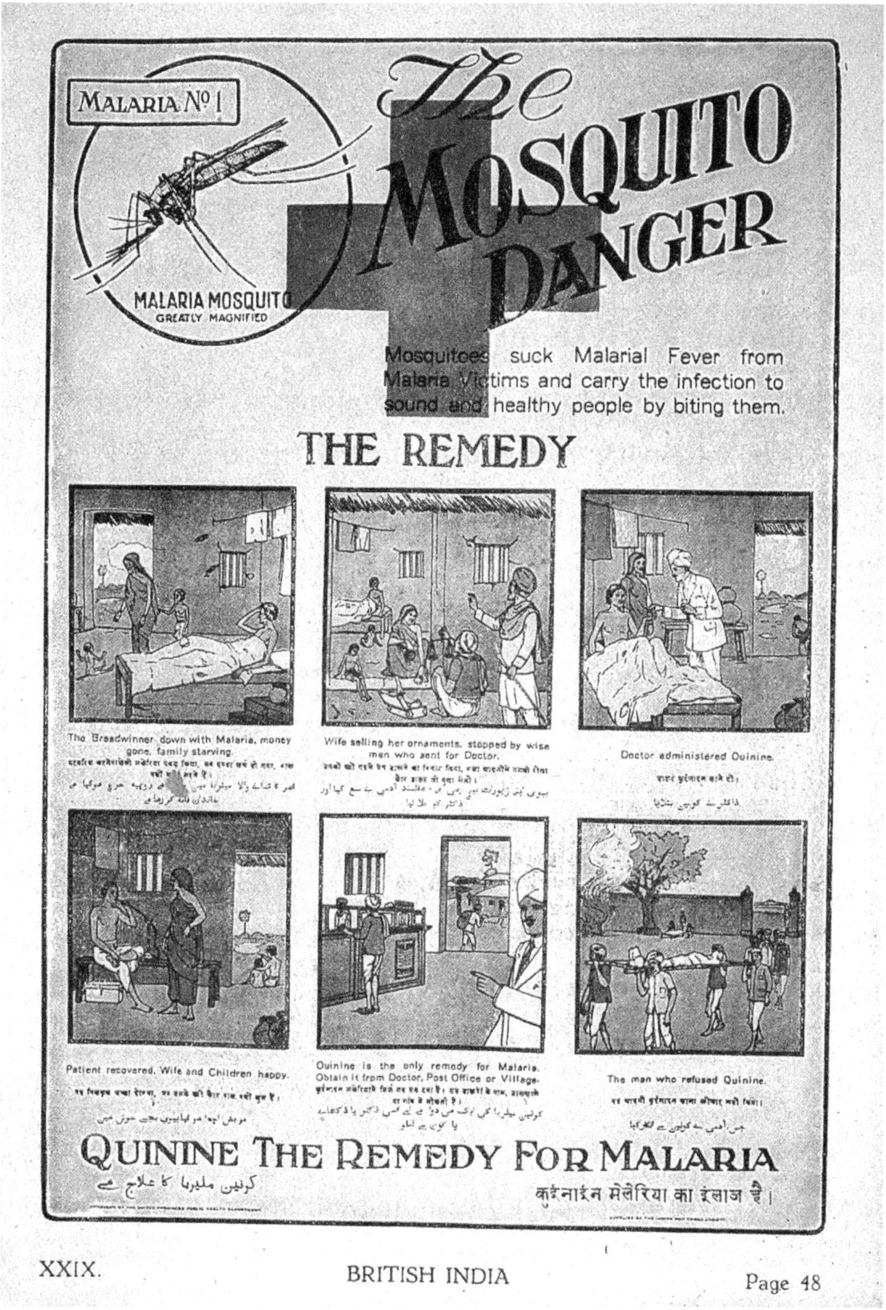

Figure A-2: *A publication in British-controlled India in 1927 emphasizes 'Quinine the remedy for malaria'. The panel at the lower right shows a funeral procession, with the caption 'The man who refused quinine'. Malaria was responsible for 150-300 million deaths worldwide during the 20th century. In the U.S., The Office of Malaria Control in War Areas was established in 1942 in Atlanta, in view of the illnesses' prevalence in the American south, and later grew into the Center for Disease Control and Prevention (CDC).*

Syphilis, the 'great pox', and its aftermath, dementia paralytica

The geographic origins of syphilis continue to be debated; one popular belief is that it was brought back to the Old World by Columbus' crew, while others argue that it already existed on both continents, perhaps unrecognized, from a much earlier time. The sixteenth century Swiss physician Paracelsus (Mendelson, 2020a) colorfully described it as the result of a liaison between a prostitute and a French leper. Regardless of its origin, it rapidly spread across Europe in the late 1400s and 1500s, often in the trail of various armies, beginning with the taking of Naples by the French in 1495. It carried a variety of names, including 'the French disease' in Italy, 'the Spanish disease' in the Netherlands, and 'the great pox' (as opposed to smallpox) in Britain.

Initially, syphilis was a much more acute and fulminant illness than we know today, presumably because it was new, or at least a new form of an older disease, for the population. It was manifest as skin lesions over most of the body, and was often fatal within a few months. Over the centuries, it became a somewhat milder, endemic disease as resistance may have developed and less virulent strains of the bacterium *Treponema pallidum* became more common. What was not realized until some time later was that the bacterium could persist in the body for decades, and reappear much later in the form of a psychiatric and neurological disorder.

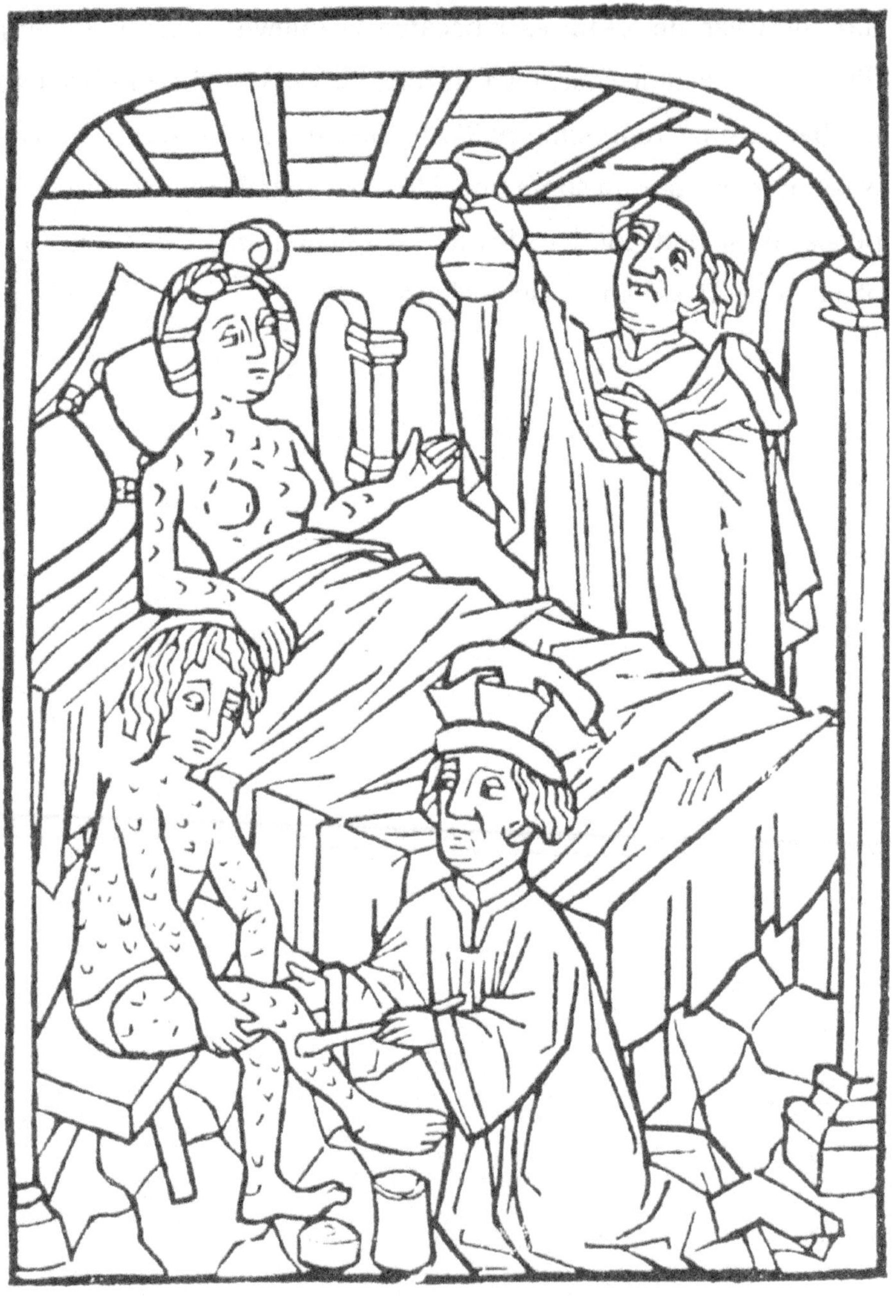

Figure A-3: *This 1498 drawing from Vienna shows the skin lesions of syphilis being treated with mercury.*

Dementia paralytica (general paresis of the insane or GPI) was first recognized as a distinct illness in the asylums of Paris during the years of the Napoleonic wars, and soon reports from other European countries began to appear as well. It was thought to reflect a weakness found in dissolute characters. As early as 1857 the German physicians Friedrich von Esmarch and Peter Willers Jessen had suggested that dementia paralytica might be due to syphilis, and the suspicion grew throughout the century. It was not until after 1905, though, when the spirochete bacterium causing syphilis had been identified by Fritz Schaudinn and Erich Hoffmann, and then later in 1913 when Hideyo Noguchi found them in the nervous systems of patients, that this became conclusive. Dementia paralytica then came to be understood to be a form of meningoencephalitis (a disorder of the brain and its covering tissues) resulting in atrophy of the cerebral hemispheres, particularly the frontal and temporal lobes.

Dementia paralytica is found in about seven percent of persons with syphilis, and generally appears 10-30 years after contracting it. At first the symptoms are vague, involving insomnia, headaches and fatigue. As it progresses there may be personality changes, impulsive or asocial behavior, depressed mood, or manic symptoms. Memory disturbances, difficulty thinking, and confusion become evident, as do delusions, often with qualities of megalomania (for instance, false beliefs of being royalty or god-like). Neurological symptoms such as tremors, overactive muscular reflexes, difficulty speaking, and paralyses typically develop. Patients often develop a characteristic gait in which the feet seem to slap the ground, due to a loss of sensation. Some learn to minimize this by looking at their feet as they walk. Unlike in other kinds of psychoses, there is a very characteristic reflex of the pupils, in which they become very small when focusing on a near object, but not when exposed to a bright light (the 'Argyll Robertson pupil'). Gradually there is weight loss and wasting of the musculature accompanying the mental deterioration, and sometimes almost continual seizures ('status epilepticus') with almost invariably lethal consequences.

Wagner-Jauregg was aware that in rare cases, some patients did recover. Retrospectively (in his Nobel Prize paper in 1927) he said that he had taken to heart the teaching of Francis Bacon, the sixteenth century English philosopher, who said that it was of the utmost importance to examine the rare times when a basically incurable illness got better. He and others observed that in these exceptional situations, the recovering patient often had experienced an illness producing fever, and this became one of the foundations of the febrile therapy he subsequently developed. It was reinforced by his finding that among those to whom he gave tuberculin, those with more lasting benefits had often later experienced some other febrile illness.

At the time that Wagner-Jauregg began studying febrile therapy with tuberculin in the 1890s, there was little else available, aside from mercury and to some degree iodine. Their rate of success was low, though never firmly established until 1914, when a case series by

Runge-Kiel found that among untreated patients remissions appeared in 3.9%, increasing to 9.3% with iodine and 11.4% with mercury (Wagner-Jauregg, 1927).

Shortly after his co-discovery of the spirochete bacteria causing syphilis, the dermatologist Erich Hoffmann noted their resemblance to the trypanosomes which produce sleeping sickness. He encouraged the German physician Paul Ehrlich to see if a drug similar to those effective against trypanosomes might be useful for syphilis. Ehrlich used as a starting point the organic arsenic drug Atoxyl, and by 1910 came up with Salvarsan, 'the arsenic that saves', followed by Neosalvarsan in 1912 (Mendelson, 2020b). They represented a major step forward in treating the acute phases of syphilis, but were of little benefit by themselves in dementia paralytica. Thus the stage was set for the widespread enthusiasm when Wagner-Jauregg introduced malaria therapy after 1917.

Tuberculosis, the 'white plague'

Its role in this narrative:

During the nineteenth century, tuberculosis (TB) had reached epidemic proportions, and may have been responsible for one quarter of the deaths in Europe (Saleem and Azher, 2013). In the 1880s, by some estimates almost one in seven Germans succumbed to it. Tuberculosis appears at a number of places in the events described here. Wagner-Jauregg suffered from it in his student years. In Chapter Two, we mentioned that it was while caring for her father's terminal tuberculosis that Bertha Pappenheim's hysterical symptoms first appeared. Wagner-Jauregg's mother died from tuberculosis when he was 10, as did Freud's mother during her old age in 1930.

Tuberculosis was known as 'the white plague', and though it was observed to be more common in poorer and more crowded areas, its cause was unknown. It was not until 1869 that Jean-Antoine Villemin at the Val-de-Grâce hospital in Paris demonstrated its infectious nature by producing the illness in rabbits who had been injected with material from infected humans. It also occupies an interesting spot in the history of medicine in that another Parisian physician, René Laennec, who was also a skilled musician and made his own flutes, created the stethoscope in his efforts to study TB earlier in the century. (He later died at age 45 of the illness he was studying.)

Tuberculin:

In 1882, Robert Koch, a German physician and bacteriologist, demonstrated that it was an infectious disease caused by the microorganism *Mycobacterium tuberculosis,* and in 1890 announced that he had developed a treatment, tuberculin, which was a glycerin extract of proteins from the bacteria.

The initial enthusiasm for tuberculin was widespread, and this was the point at which Wagner-Jauregg learned about it. His interest arose from the notion that it might produce the desired fever without the hazards of introducing an infectious disease to a patient. Clinics were opening throughout Europe, often in a celebratory spirit. As the next year or two went by, however, it became clear that its effectiveness in treating tuberculosis had been greatly over-rated. A study of 1769 patients in 1891 reported cures in only 1%, while 34% got slightly better, 55% had minimal effect, and 4% died presumably due to the underlying tuberculosis (Huebner et al., 1993).

It also turned out that subcutaneous injection with tuberculin as performed in those years was far from benign. From the beginning it had been recognized that for several hours it was likely to produce fever, accompanied by joint pains and nausea. Later more severe reactions were reported and even deaths were attributed to the treatment. When questioned, Koch revealed that he had tested it on himself and his then 16-year-old mistress (and later wife) Hedwig Freiberg. He was unable to produce the results of the extensive animal testing which he claimed to have done. The final straw came when the renowned pathologist Rudolf Virchow performed autopsies showing live bacteria in tuberculin-treated patients, and even found evidence that the treatment may have stimulated previously latent bacteria. As described in Chapter Three, Wagner-Jauregg stopped its use, though he resumed a few years later in Vienna, by which time a more benign dosage and procedure had been determined.

Not surprisingly, the days of tuberculin as a treatment for tuberculosis rapidly came to an end, but it lives on in another capacity under the name of purified protein derivative (PPD). Koch had also advocated its administration as a way of testing for prior exposure to TB bacteria, and the technique was later refined by others including Charles Mantoux in 1912. A small amount of tuberculin is injected between the skin layers (intradermally) of the forearm; between 48-72 hours later, a person with bacterial exposure will show evidence of an immune reaction, as seen by induration (a hard, raised area) and redness. In the case of a positive test, further procedures are then needed to determine if the person has latent TB or active illness.

Freud and antisemitism

The role of Freud's Jewish background in his career is a complex topic and the subject of many scholarly works (for instance, Frosh, 2004); it goes well beyond the scope of this book, which is focused on his relationship with Wagner-Jauregg. Here are just a few brief comments about how his Jewish heritage interacted with two of the topics we've touched on:

Freud's relation to Charcot.

Freud's training with Charcot involving the use of hypnosis and hysteria marked the beginning of his belief that there might be a level of mental activity not available to the conscious mind (Chapter Two). Another aspect of this period, however, was that Charcot was very interested in the hereditary aspects of illnesses. He frequently made the point that hysteria, arthritis, and some neurological conditions appeared more frequently in Jewish populations, which in Europe at the time were often relatively closed communities and prone to endogamy (marriage within a social group). Although many, including Charcot's son (Goldstein, 1985) made it clear that he was not antisemitic, others such as the neurologist Henry Meige and the journalist Edouard Drumont frequently quoted his work in their antisemitic writings, in which they emphasized the mythical character of the 'Wandering Jew'. The prominence of the issue of French antisemitism as seen in the Dreyfus affair of 1894 has led many to look at possible antecedents in the previous decades, but it seems more likely that Charcot's own interest, though later misused by others, was a genuine one of exploring genetic influences on psychiatric illness.

Charcot's assertions about the possibly higher rate of certain illnesses in Jewish communities may, however, have had an affect on Freud. It has been speculated that it led to a cooling of his relationship with Charcot, and that it even may have influenced Freud's movement away from hereditary factors in favor of sexual trauma in the genesis of hysteria (Roth, 2008). Charcot also did not share Freud's fascination with the case of Breuer's patient Bertha Pappenheim (Chapter Two), which perhaps also may have led to some distancing.

Antisemitism in Viennese academe.

In Chapter Five, we touched on Freud's remarkably slow rise in the academic community compared to Wagner-Jauregg, and commented on the many reasons involved. It seems likely that antisemitism was among them, though the degree to which it played a role is hard to know.

In the 1960s, J. and R. Glickhorn, husband-and-wife historians, argued that it was Freud's character which was the major factor hindering him. They pointed to what they viewed as his excessive interest in money, his missing many lectures, and a disagreeable manner. Whitrow (1993) responded to these comments, noting for instance that Freud came from a financially stressed background, so that financial security might reasonably be a concern for him, and quoting an 1896 report indicating that he had faithfully given lectures regularly for the 20 preceding semesters. The psychoanalyst Kurt Eissler, defended Freud as well, suggesting that the Glickhorns' work amounted to an effort to unrealistically vindicate the university (Eissler, 1966), which according to a contemporary account had a long history of antisemitism (Kniefacz, 2020). As but one example, in 1876, while Freud and Wagner-Jauregg were studying at the University of Vienna, Theodor Billroth, a faculty member and perhaps the most famous surgeon in Europe, published a book on German education that was very nationalistic and highly critical of Jewish students (Buklijas, 2007). Though controversial in liberal circles, it was quickly embraced by student groups, and is often cited in the history of Austrian antisemitism. Even in his earliest years there, Freud could hardly have failed to aware of this movement at the institution with which he was to be affiliated for most of his life.

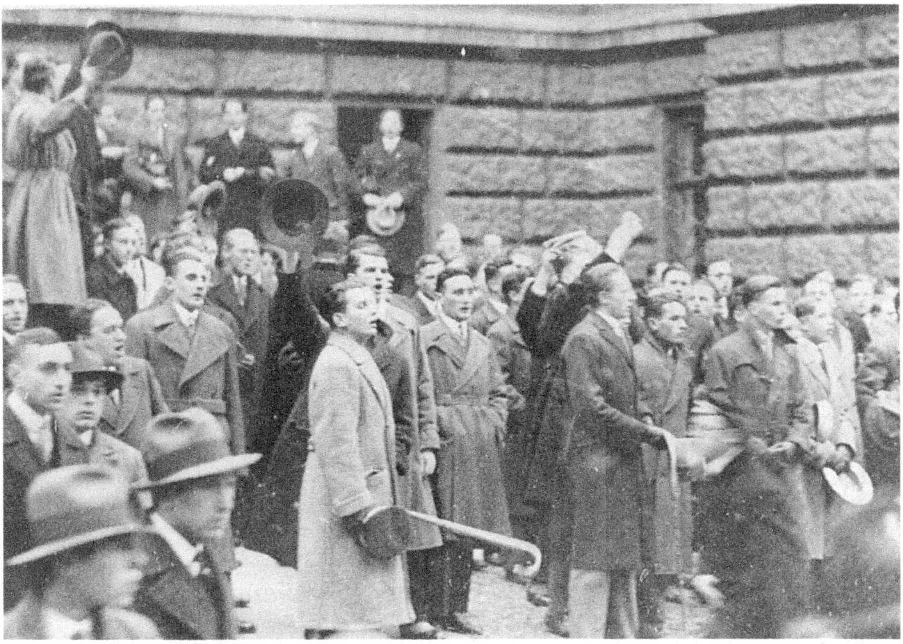

Figure A-4: *A protest against a Nazi effort to exclude enrollment of new Jewish students at the University of Vienna, 1938.*

Though the influence of antisemitism on Freud's academic career is a matter of debate, its effect on his later life was dramatic. As described in Chapter Four, the growing antisemitic sentiment in the 1920s led him to reconsider his identity with German culture. His books were burned in 1933, and in 1938 he was persecuted by the Gestapo, and was forced to flee to London.

REFERENCES for APPENDIX

Buklijas, T.: Surgery and national identity in late nineteenth-century Vienna. Std. Hist. Philos. Biol. Biomed Sci. 38: 756-774, 2007. https://www.ncbi.nlm.nih.gov/pmc/articles/PMC2605547/

CDC: Malaria, 2019. https://www.cdc.gov/malaria/about/disease.html (Accessed February 21, 2022).

Eissler, K. R. (1966) *Sigmund Freud und die Wiener Universitiit.* Ueber die Pseudo-Wissenschaftlichkeit der jiingsten Freud Biographik. Bern and Stuttgart: Huber.

Frosh, S.: Freud, psychoanalysis and anti-semitism. Psychoanalytic Review 91: 309-330, 2004. https://psycnet.apa.org/record/2004-18333-001

Glickhorn, J. & R.: *Sigmund Freud's akademische Laufbahn.* Vienna and Innsbruck: Urban and Schwarzenberg, 1960.

Goldstein, J.: The wandering Jew and the problem of psychiatric anti-semitism in fin-de-siecle France. J. Contemporary History 20: 521-552, 1985.
https://www.jstor.org/stable/260396

Huebner, R.E.; Schein, M.F.; and Bass, J.B.: The tuberculin skin test. Clin. Infectious Dis. 17: 968-975, 1993.
https://www.jstor.org/stable/4457498

Jones, E.: *Sigmund Freud Life and Work, 1961, p. 233.*

Kniefacz, K.: A dark history: anti-semitism at the University of Vienna. Austrian Press & Information Service in the United States: New Austrian Information, Vol. 71, 2020.
https://www.austrianinformation.org/fall-2015/dark-history
(Accessed February 20, 2022).

Mendelson, W.B.: *Nepenthe's Children: The History of the Discoveries of Medicines for Sleep and Anesthesia.* Pythagoras Press, 2020a.
https://www.amazon.com/dp/B08H4XDZBN

Mendelson, W.B.: *Molecules, Madness, and Malaria: How Victorian Fabric Dyes Evolved into Modern Medicines for Mental Illness and Infectious Disease.* Pythagoras Press, 2020b.
https://www.amazon.com/dp/B088QPG14K

Roth, E.: Hysteria, heredity and anti-semitism: Freud's quiet rebellion. Psychoanalysis and history. 10: 149-168, 2008.
https://www.euppublishing.com/doi/full/10.3366/E1460823508000147

Saleem, A. and Azher, M.: The next pandemic—tuberculosis: the oldest disease of mankind rising one more time. Brit. J. Med. Practitioners. 6(1): a615, 2013.
https://www.bjmp.org/files/2013-6-2/bjmp-2013-6-2-a615.pdf
(Accessed Feb 18, 2022).

PICTURE CREDITS

The author's assessment is that all images are in the public domain or presented under the terms of Section 107 of the U.S. Copyright Law (the 'Fair Use' provision), and in one case, under commercial license.. When appropriate, all reasonable efforts have been employed to trace copyright holders and to get their permission for the use of copyright material. The author apologizes for any errors or omissions in this list and will gratefully include any corrections in future editions if notified.

Cover illustration:

Top: (Freud's couch). Robert Huffstutter, in Wikimedia Commons, under Creative Commons Attribution 2.0 license.

Bottom: (fever thermometer). Franz van Duns in Wikimedia Commons, under Creative Commons Attribution-Share Alike 4.0 International license. Design of overall illustration by Russell Rosenberg, PhD.

Figure 1-1: (University of Vienna). © Hubertl in Wikimedia Commons ,under the Creative Commons Attribution-Share Alike 4.0 International License.

Figure 1-3: (Stricker, motor end plate). W.Englemann, Leipzig, in Wellcome Collection, Creative Commons Attribution 4.0 International License.

Figure 1-4: (postage stamp of Wagner-Jauregg). Stamp issued by Austria in 1957. From Mostphotos.com, under commercial license.

Figure 1- 5 (Seven Viennese Doctors, including Wagner-Jauregg). Seven Viennese doctors, artist's signature indistinct. Process print, 1913.Wellcome Collection, Creative Commons Attribution 4.0 International License; per Holly Peel, Image Services Manager on March 9. 2022.

Figure 2-1: (16 year old Freud). Author unknown, in Wikimedia Commons, which states 'This work is in the public domain in its country of origin and other countries and areas where the copyright term is the author's life plus 70 years or fewer.'

Figure 2-2: (Meynert brain dissection). Theodor Meynert in Wikimedia Commons, which states 'This work is in the public domain in its country of origin and other countries and areas where the copyright term is the author's life plus 70 years or fewer.'

Figure 2-3: (Charcot). Jean-Martin Charcot demonstrating hysteria in a hypnotised patient at the Salpêtrière. Etching by A. Lurat, 1888, after P.A.A. Brouillet, 1887. From the Wellcome Collection, under Attribution 4.0 International (CC BY 4.0) license.

Figure 2-4: (topographic and structural models). Historicair, in Wikimedia Commons, which quotes 'I, the copyright holder of this work, release this work into the public domain. This applies worldwide. In some countries this may not be legally possible; if so: *I grant anyone the right to use this work for any purpose, without any conditions, unless such conditions are required by law.'*

Figure 2-5: (Freud and Followers). Photograph, 1909 (gift of Mr. Ernst Freud) in the Wellcome Collection, under Creative Commons Attribution 4.0 International License.

Figure 2-6: (Ten Viennese Doctors, including Freud). Noorden, C.V., contributor: Process print, 1913. Wellcome Collection, under Creative Commons Attribution 4.0 International License.

Figure 3-1: (medical transport barge). Medicine during the First World War - Medical Transport. British official photographer, in Wikimedia Commons, which states 'This image was created and released by the Imperial War Museum on the IWM Non Commercial Licence. Photographs taken, or artworks created, by a member of the forces during their active service duties are covered by Crown Copyright provisions. Faithful reproductions may be reused under that licence, which is considered expired 50 years after their creation.'

Figure 3-2: (galvanic therapy in the 18th century). Colored etching in the Wellcome Collection, under Creative Commons Attribution 4.0 International License.

Figure 3-3: (superego, ego and id). Meerabsolomon, in Wikimedia Commons, creative Commons-Share Alike 4.0 International License.

Figure 3-4: (Al Capone). Pennsylvania Department of Corrections/FBI, in Wikimedia Commons, which states 'This image or file is a work of a Federal Bureau of Investigation employee, take or made as part of that person's official duties. As a work of the U.S. federal government, the image is in the public domain in the United States.'

Figure 3-5: (hypertherm). Uncredited WPA photographer, in Wikimedia Commons, which states ' This work is in the public domain in the United States because it is a work prepared by an officer or employee of the Unites States government as part of that person's official duties under the terms of Title 17, Chapter 1, Section 105 of the US Code.

Figure 4-1: (Nazi book burning). Office of Emergency Management, Office of War Information, in Wikimedia Commons, which states 'This file was provided to Wikimedia Commons by the National Archives and Records Administration as part of a cooperation project. The National Archives and Records Administration provides images depicting American and global history which are public domain or licensed under a free license.'

Figure 5-1: (Freud and Wagner-Jauregg portraits.).

LEFT: (Freud) Max Halberstadt, in Wikimedia Commons, which states 'This work is in the public domain in the United States because it was published (or registered with the U.S. Copyright Office) before January 1, 1927.

RIGHT: (Wagner Jauregg, cropped) Unknown author, in Wikimedia Commons, which states 'This work is in the public domain in its country of origin and other countries and areas where the copyright term is the author's life plus 70 years or fewer.' Design of overall illustration by Russell Rosenberg, PhD.

Figure 5-2: (Wagner-Jauregg and staff). Anonymous, in Wikimedia Commons, which states 'This work is in the public domain in its country of origin and other countries and areas where the copyright term is the author's life plus 70 years or fewer'.

Figure A-1: (fever patterns). Jack Edelbrock in Wikimedia Commons, under Creative Commons Attribution-Share Alike 4.0 International License.

Figure A-2: (quinine). Malaria and qunine. Bureau for Increasing Use of Quinine, Amsterdam, 1927, in the Wellcome Collection, under Creative Commons Attribution 4.0 International License.

Figure A-3: (syphilis) Meerabsolomon, in Wikimedia Commons, under Creative Commons-Share Alike 4.0 International License.

Figure A-4: (Protest at University of Vienna). 'Students riot at the University of Vienna after Nazi attempt to prevent Jews from entering the university'. Unknown author, in Wikimedia Commons, which states 'This work is considered in the public domain in the United States because its copyright was owned or administered by the Alien Property Custodian and the copyright in the source country is or was owned by a government or instrumentality thereof. The above provision is contained in 17 USC 104A(a)(2).'

BIBLIOGRAPHIC NOTE

Portions of the text on the effect of World War I on Freud's thinking (in Chapter Three), and of the period leading to World War II (in Chapter Four), were adapted from the Prologue in *Trial by Fire: World War II and the Founders of Modern Neuroscience and Psychopharmacology* (Mendelson, W.B., Pythagoras Press, 2021), and here are addressed more fully.

ACKNOWLEDGEMENT

The author appreciates the skilled work of Russell Rosenberg PhD in the design of the cover illustration and Figure 5.1.

Made in the USA
Monee, IL
05 November 2026

67843126R00075